The Wellness Code for Vibrant Ageing

Unleash Your Full Potential: To Celebrate Ageing as a Journey of Growth, Transformation, and Fulfillment

Uma Gupta

(M.Sc Foods & Nutrition)

ABOUT THE AUTHOR

**Mrs. Uma Gupta,
Author of "The Wellness Code for Vibrant Ageing."**

Mrs. Uma Gupta, M. Sc. (Food & Nutrition) is an eminent Health and Wellness Coach, an Energy Healer, is dedicated to empowering health seekers with knowledge and strategies to elevate wellness and transform lives to live healthy, happy, prosperous and spiritually fulfilled lives. She strongly recommends each soul to live a purposeful life, integrated with their values and vision and with a heart full of love❤

DEDICATION

This book is dedicated to all the seniors who are ready to celebrate a journey of growth, transformation, and fulfillment. Special dedication to my Father-in-law, Late Sh. Prem Nath Gupta Ji, Pita Ji, and my husband Late Dr. Amit Gupta who are my true heroes. They lived their journey of growth, transformation, and fulfillment with a resilient and positive mindset. Despite inevitable health challenges, they completed their journey serving the community till a week before their final retirement from the journey of life.

"You only live once, but if you do it right, once is enough."—
Mae West

ACKNOWLEDGEMENT

Writing this book has been a journey filled with countless moments of inspiration, support, and encouragement from many incredible individuals.

First and foremost, I extend my deepest gratitude to my parents, my children, and my siblings for their unwavering love, understanding, and patience throughout this endeavor. Your belief in me has been my greatest source of strength.

I am indebted to my mentors Dr. M.S. Manjunath, Dr. Inderjit Aggarwal, R. Lakshmi Dhevi, and advisors, whose guidance and wisdom have shaped my thinking and enriched this work in profound ways. Your insights have been invaluable.

I also want to express my appreciation to the numerous experts and researchers whose work laid the foundation for the ideas explored in this book. Your contributions to the field are immeasurable.

To my friends and colleagues who provided encouragement, feedback, and moral support along the way, thank you for believing in me and cheering me on.

Finally, I extend heartfelt thanks to the readers who will embark on this journey with me. Your curiosity and open-mindedness inspire me to continue exploring, learning, and sharing.

This book is a testament to the collective effort of all who have touched my life. Thank you for being a part of this journey.

FOREWORD

Mathew Cherian
Global Ambassador of Ageing
HelpAge International and
Former CEO, HelpAge India

It is indeed a great pleasure for me to write the Foreword for Uma Gupta's book on "The Wellness Code for Vibrant Ageing." Uma Gupta has written her personal experiences and advances made in Health and Well Being and advances in the current state of Ageing. She has attempted to make one's life richer and graceful and she has coined the word "Vibrant Ageing" which is a step ahead of Active Ageing combines the body, mind and spirit. Uma is a well know nutritionist and wellness coach and advice both young and the old.

It is heartening to note that her immense knowledge and experience has been distilled to bring out valuable pearls of wisdom, compiled into a common code which is easy to understand and practice for a vibrant positive Life. The pace of ageing in India and increased longevity means that most Indians will cross 80 years of age and women blessed with stronger genetics will live much, much longer.

How can we apply the Code for Vibrant Ageing to make our lives graceful, happier and more fulfilling. The book is timely and opportune for many of us working in the Field of Ageing as we celebrate the "WHO decade for Healthy Ageing with the motto of "Leave no one behind".

Integrating the body, mind and spirit in the pursuit of wellness, her advice on pursuing meditation and the method of integrating the spirit in our lives is to seek the "power of now" and transform ourselves as we age. Some of the case studies have a transformative experience in understanding the code. Her basic principles of Healthy Eating, the benefits of Physical Activity and Nurturing Social Connections, along with deep meditation. She explores the science and impact of breathing known for centuries in Yoga as "Pranayama." The Social Connections for the Old and the young in the fast-paced modern life will help counter the isolation and loneliness felt in later life. These practical tips and principles help the reader in the pathway to lead a vibrant life.

Uma Gupta's personal experience and practical knowledge has produced an insightful compendium for older persons so that the code can lead to a blissful life full of joy and happiness. As a first source book on Vibrant Ageing in India, it will be valuable resource both for the Young and the Old so that it becomes a purpose driven set of objectives and help us to work hard to live in inner peace and harmony. The elixir of life is not a magical potion to drink but resides within all of us. It is upto each one of us to search for this magical code within us and the book will help us in the path. Uma Gupta's book is a must read for unlocking our own code for living a vibrant life and "unleash your own potential."

Mathew Cherian
Global Ambassador of Ageing
HelpAge International and
Former CEO, HelpAge India

Contents

Overview of the Book's Purpose and Objectives

"The Wellness Code for Vibrant Ageing: Unleash Your Full Potential" is a comprehensive guide designed to empower seniors in their Golden years to embrace Ageing with vitality, purpose, and well-being.

According to a WHO report, the pace of population Ageing is much faster than in the past, but the proportion of life in good health has remained broadly constant, implying that the additional years are spent in poor health. If people can experience these extra years of life in good health and if they live in a supportive environment, their ability to do the things they value will be little different. The greater purpose of this book is to empower readers to live these additional years in good health and be more productive to themselves and to the community.

People worldwide are living longer. Today, most people can expect to live into their sixties and beyond. Every country in the world is experiencing growth in both the size and the proportion of older persons in the population.

By 2030, 1 in 6 people in the world will be aged 60 years or over. At this time, the share of the population aged 60 years and over will increase from 1 billion in 2020 to 1.4 billion. By 2050, the world's population of people aged 60 years and older will double (2.1 billion). The number of persons aged 80 years or older is expected to triple between 2020 and 2050 to reach 426 million.

A longer life brings with it opportunities, not only for older people and their families but also for societies as a whole. Additional years provide the chance to pursue new activities such as further education, a new career, or a long-neglected passion. Older people also contribute in many ways to their families and communities. Yet the extent of these opportunities and contributions depends heavily on one factor: health.

Although some of the variations in older people's health are genetic, most is due to people's physical and social environments – including their homes, neighborhoods, and communities. Maintaining healthy behavior throughout life, particularly eating a balanced diet, engAgeing in regular physical activity, and refraining from tobacco use, all contribute to reducing the risk of non-communicable diseases, improving physical and mental capacity, and delaying care dependency.

Supportive physical and social environments also enable people to do what is important to them, despite losses in capacity. The availability of safe and accessible public buildings and transport, and places that are easy to walk around, are examples of supportive environments. In developing a public-health response to Ageing, it is important not just to consider individual and environmental approaches that ameliorate the losses associated with older age, but also those that may reinforce recovery, adaptation, and psychological and social growth.

WHO Response

The United Nations (UN) General Assembly declared 2021–2030 the UN Decade of Healthy Ageing and asked WHO to lead the implementation. The UN Decade of Healthy Ageing is a global collaboration bringing together governments, civil society, international agencies, professionals, academia, the media, and the private sector for 10 years of concerted, catalytic, and collaborative action to foster longer and healthier lives.

The UN Decade of Healthy Ageing (2021–2030) seeks to reduce health inequities and improve the lives of older people, their families, and communities through collective action in four areas: changing how we think, feel, and act towards age and ageism; developing communities in ways that foster the abilities of older people; delivering person-centered integrated care and primary health services responsive to older people; and providing older people who need it with access to quality long-term care.

Key Facts

All countries face major challenges to ensure that their health and social systems are ready to make the most of this demographic shift.

The pace of population Ageing is much faster than in the past.

In 2020, the number of people aged 60 years and older outnumbered children younger than 5 years.

Between 2015 and 2050, the proportion of the world's population over 60 years will nearly double from 12% to 22%.

Let Us Understand the Purpose of the Book

Grounded in the principles of holistic wellness, the book offers practical strategies, expert insights, and inspirational guidance to help seniors unlock their full potential and live their best lives in later years. It's all about our attitude towards how we wish to live our life, the golden opportunity our soul is blessed with in this life to express itself in a fruitful manner, not merely living days, months, and years.

Living life with a purpose infuses us with boundless enthusiasm and joy. Aging vibrantly is to fill the treasure of life with pearls of wisdom gained from our experiences, which may be filled with success or challenges. With a positive mindset, we explore our potential to move forward effectively, focused on our actions. It is more than walking on the road shown by Google Map. It's for us to follow the compass directed by our values and wisdom to make wiser choices, living life to excellence with boundless enthusiasm integrated with our vision and with a heart full of love and compassion.

The purpose of this book is to challenge common myths and misconceptions about aging and empower seniors with the knowledge, tools, and resources they need to thrive in their later years.

By appreciating aging as a natural and enriching phase of life, the book aims to inspire readers to adopt a proactive approach to their health and well-being, cultivate resilience, and embrace the opportunities for growth and personal development that come with age.

Objectives of the book are:

1. Empowerment: The book aims to empower seniors to take charge of their health and well-being by providing them with motivation, practical strategies, actionable advice, and evidence-based information to make informed decisions about their wellness journey starting much before they complete the first half-century of life.

2. Education: By debunking myths and misconceptions about aging, the book seeks to educate readers about the potential for growth, fulfillment, and transformation in later life. Through engaging storytelling, expert insights, and real-life examples, readers gain a deeper understanding of the aging process and the factors that contribute to vibrant aging.

3. Inspiration: The book aims to inspire readers to cultivate a positive mindset, embrace change, and approach aging with optimism and enthusiasm. Through stories of resilience, personal anecdotes, and motivational messages, readers are encouraged to unleash their full potential and live their lives to the fullest.

4. Practical Guidance: Practicality is at the core of the book's objectives, offering readers actionable strategies, tips, and exercises to incorporate into their daily lives. From nutrition and exercise to stress management and social connections, the book provides practical

guidance for seniors to enhance their physical, mental, and emotional well-being.

5. Support: Lastly, the book aims to provide support and encouragement to seniors as they navigate the challenges and opportunities of aging. By offering resources, support networks, and a sense of community, the book fosters a supportive environment where seniors can share their experiences, learn from others, and feel empowered to live their best lives in later years.

By aligning with these objectives, "The Wellness Code for Vibrant Aging" serves as a comprehensive resource and companion for seniors on their journey to aging with vitality, purpose, and well-being.

1

LET US UNDERSTAND WHAT'S VIBRANT AGING

"The Wellness Code for Vibrant Ageing: Unleash Your Full Potential" takes you on a journey into the art of Ageing with vitality, purpose, and well-being. Within these pages, we embark on a transformative exploration of what it truly means to embrace the golden years with enthusiasm, resilience, and a zest for life. Indeed, we are filled with gratitude for being blessed with an opportunity to play our role on this planet Earth and contribute our bit towards promoting the Golden Age.

Ageing often carries a negative connotation, perceived as a time of decline marked by limitations, losses, and diminishing capacities. Yet, contrary to popular belief, the later years of life hold immense potential for growth, fulfillment, and personal development.

Vibrant Ageing transcends mere survival; it embodies a philosophy of thriving – physically, mentally, emotionally, and spiritually, regardless of age. But what exactly is vibrant Ageing, and how can we cultivate it in our own lives?

Vibrant Ageing is more than just the absence of illness; it's a holistic approach to wellness that encompasses every aspect of our being. It's about nurturing our physical health through nourishing nutrition, regular exercise, breathing exercises like pranayama, and preventive healthcare. It's about fostering mental and emotional well-being through resilience, a positive mindset, and meaningful social connections. It's about accepting the inevitable and embracing change, finding purpose, and living with intention and authenticity. It's about having the zest to serve with empathy, exploring the power of synergy within the societal web.

In essence, vibrant Ageing is about unleashing our full potential – tapping into our inner reserves of strength, wisdom, self-discipline, mindset, and vitality to create a life that is rich in meaning, purpose, and joy. It's about getting connected with our inner sovereign self, exploring our hidden talents, and nurturing them to serve mankind and add greater value to life.

> *"The purpose of life is not to simply be happy. It is to*
> *be useful, to be honorable, to be compassionate, to have it*
> *make some difference that you have lived and lived well."*
> *- Ralph Waldo Emerson*

Throughout this book, we'll explore the principles and practices of vibrant Ageing, expert insights, and personal anecdotes to guide us on this transformative journey. We'll challenge common myths and misconceptions about Ageing, and we'll provide practical strategies, actionable advice, and inspirational stories to empower you to live your best life in later years.

So, whether you're embarking on the adventure of Ageing yourself or supporting a loved one on their journey, I invite you to join me as we discover the keys to vibrant Ageing – keys that will unlock a world of possibilities, opportunities, and fulfillment in the golden years ahead.

Vibrant Ageing is Ageing with Grace and Embracing the Beauty of Life's Seasons.

Let us learn from Janki's experience, who lived in a small village in Uttarakhand on the foothills of the Himalayan mountains.

Janki was a beloved member of the community, known for her warmth, kindness, and unwavering optimism. As she gracefully navigated her later years, Janki embodied the true essence of Ageing with grace. From her cozy cottage adorned with colorful flowers and a kitchen garden in the backyard to her welcoming smile that lit up the room, Janki radiated a sense of inner peace and contentment that seemed to defy the passage of time. Despite the inevitable changes and challenges that came with Ageing, Janki embraced each new day as a precious gift, cherishing the beauty and richness of life's seasons. Her luminous nature attracted people towards her.

One sunny afternoon, as Janki sat on her porch sipping warm water infused with Himalayan herbs and admiring the vibrant hues of the blooming flowers, she was visited by a young couple from the village. Priya and Nitheesh, newlyweds with dreams of starting a family, had come seeking Janki's wisdom and guidance on Ageing with grace.

"Please, won't you share your secret with us, Amma?" Priya asked, her eyes filled with curiosity and admiration. "How do you remain so radiant and joyful despite the passing years?"

Janki smiled warmly and beckoned the young couple to join her on the porch. As they settled into their chairs, Janki offered them the aromatic herbal infusion and began to weave a tale of wisdom and inspiration, sharing her reflections on Ageing with grace as a blissful journey of self-discovery and growth.

"My dear friends," Janki began, "Ageing is not something to be feared or resisted, but rather embraced as a natural and beautiful part of life's journey. Each passing year brings with it new experiences, wisdom, and opportunities for growth."

She went on to explain how she had learned to cultivate a mindset of gratitude, acceptance, and resilience in the face of Ageing. Instead of lamenting the wrinkles on her face or the aches in her bones, Janki chose to focus on the blessings and joys that surrounded her each day—the laughter of children playing in the village square, the gentle caress of the breeze against her skin, the warmth of friendship and community.

"As we age, we are gifted with the opportunity to deepen our connections, savor life's simple pleasures, and embrace the fullness of who we are," Janki continued. "It is a time to let go of the pressures of youth and embrace the wisdom and freedom that come with age."

Priya and Nitheesh listened intently, their hearts stirred by Janki's words of wisdom and grace. Inspired by her example, they began to envision a future filled with possibilities, where Ageing was not something to be feared but celebrated as a journey of growth, transformation, and fulfillment.

As the sun began to set behind the horizon, casting a warm glow over the village, Janki bid farewell to Priya and Nitheesh, her heart brimming with gratitude and contentment. As she watched the young couple walk hand in hand down the cobblestone path, Janki knew that her words had struck a chord, igniting a spark of hope and inspiration in their hearts.

And so, dear reader, let us heed the wisdom of Janki and embrace Ageing with grace as a blissful journey of self-discovery, growth, and fulfillment. May we cherish each moment, savoring the beauty and richness of life's seasons, and embracing the fullness of who we are with open hearts and grateful spirits. Let us expand our circle of influence and act upon our concerns in a proactive manner using the knowledge and skill to make our journey graceful.

Well, the ultimate goal of Ageing healthily is to live each year and each hour full of life and enjoying this blissful gift of Life. Ageing is not losing youth but adding more pearls of wisdom from your experiences, a life lived with quality, integrated with your values, and true to your vision. The fountain of youth flows from within.

"The Fountain of Youth Within"

Once upon a time, in a small village nestled amidst rolling hills and lush greenery, there lived an elderly woman named Elena. Despite her advanced age, Elena was known throughout the village for her radiant smile, boundless energy, and unwavering zest for life. People marveled at her vitality and wondered what her secret was.

One day, a curious young traveler named Alex arrived in the village, drawn by rumors of a legendary fountain that could grant eternal youth. Determined to uncover the truth, Alex sought out Elena, hoping she could shed some light on the matter.

Elena welcomed Alex with open arms, her eyes sparkling with warmth and wisdom. Sensing his eagerness, she invited him to join her on a walk through the village, promising to share her secret along the way.

As they strolled through the cobblestone streets, Elena regaled Alex with tales of her adventurous youth – of dancing in the rain, climbing mountains, and chasing dreams with reckless abandon. She spoke of the joys and challenges she had faced, the lessons she had learned, and the moments that had shaped her into the person she was today.

With each step, Elena's spirit seemed to soar, her laughter ringing out like music in the air. Alex couldn't help but be captivated by her infectious enthusiasm and boundless energy.

Finally, as they reached the edge of the village, Elena paused and turned to Alex with a twinkle in her eye. "Here it is," she said, gesturing to the vast expanse of nature stretching out before them. "The fountain of youth you seek is not found in a distant land or hidden beneath the earth. It resides within each and every one of us – in the depths of our hearts, the power of our minds, and the resilience of our spirits."

Alex was taken aback by Elena's words, realizing that the true secret to eternal youth was not a magical elixir or mythical fountain, but a mindset – a mindset of curiosity, courage, and unwavering optimism in the face of life's challenges.

Inspired by Elena's wisdom, Alex returned to his own village with a newfound sense of purpose and determination. He vowed to live each day to the fullest, embracing every moment with gratitude and joy, knowing that the fountain of youth he sought was already within his grasp.

And so, the legend of Elena and the fountain of youth lived on, reminding all who heard it that age is but a number, and true vitality comes from within.

As for Elena, she continued to dance through life with grace and gusto, her spirit forever young and her heart forever free.

These stories illustrate the power of mindset, resilience, and a zest for life in Ageing with vitality and purpose. They encourage us to embrace each day with gratitude, curiosity, and unwavering optimism, knowing that the fountain of youth resides within our hearts and spirits.

2

─── ◆ ───

UNDERSTANDING AGING: MYTHS AND REALITIES

"Age gracefully, for it is not the passing of years that defines us, but the richness of our experiences, the depth of our character, and the resilience of our spirit." – Unknown

Ageing is a natural and inevitable part of the human experience, yet it is often shrouded in myths and misconceptions that can shape our perceptions and attitudes towards growing older. In this chapter, we will explore the truths behind Ageing, debunking common myths and uncovering the realities of this profound journey. By delving into the biological, psychological, and social aspects of Ageing, we will gain a deeper understanding of its complexities and potential for growth, fulfillment, and transformation in later life.

Debunking Common Myths and Misconceptions about Ageing:

Myth 1: Ageing is synonymous with decline and deterioration.

Reality: While it is true that Ageing can bring about physical changes and health challenges, it is not synonymous with decline. Many older adults lead active, fulfilling lives well into their later years, challenging the notion that Ageing is solely a time of deterioration. By focusing on maintaining physical and mental well-being, older adults can continue to thrive and contribute to society in meaningful ways. Many people like Pitaji are an example whom I have seen defeating this myth.

Myth 2: Memory loss and cognitive decline are inevitable with age.

Reality: While some degree of cognitive decline may occur as we age, it is not inevitable or universal. Many older adults maintain sharp cognitive function well into old age, with some even experiencing improvements in certain areas, such as wisdom and emotional intelligence. It is directly proportional to how well we nurture and use cognitive faculty. If we slow down on exercising our brain and slow down on the learning process in life, then definitely our neurons, our nerve cells like any other muscle, start undergoing atrophy. This may lead to cognitive decline. By engAgeing in mentally stimulating activities, maintaining a healthy lifestyle, continuing with learning, and sharing knowledge and wisdom, we can support brain health and preserve cognitive function to age vibrantly.

Myth 3: Older adults are technologically incompetent and resistant to change.

Reality: While older adults may have had less exposure to technology earlier in life, many are embracing digital tools and platforms to stay connected, informed, and engaged. With the rise of user-friendly devices and accessible training programs, seniors are increasingly incorporating technology into their daily lives, challenging stereotypes of technological incompetence and resistance to change. Pitaji was a live example. Though he performed excellently in his job in the recruitment department and chose to be in action even after retirement, he had a quest for learning as well. He had no exposure to digital interface technology. I remember one day when my son was demonstrating to him about how a laptop works and how you can open multiple windows/screens to work simultaneously, he very intriguingly said, "How will I close so many windows when I want to come back to the first?" But then he patiently and persistently continued learning and became an expert at it. Till a week before his ultimate retirement from life, during COVID, he was efficiently manAgeing and administering a patient service center, proactively serving so many lives by facilitating diagnostic services. So, the most important aspect is how eagerly you want something and how much effort you put into achieving your mission.

Exploring the Biological, Psychological, and Social Aspects of Ageing:

Let us understand various aspects of Ageing.

Biological Aspect: Ageing is a complex biological process influenced by a combination of genetic, environmental, and lifestyle factors. From cellular changes and hormonal fluctuations to changes in organ function and tissue integrity, Ageing affects every aspect of the body's physiology. While some age-related changes are inevitable, others can be mitigated or delayed through healthy lifestyle choices and nurturing four dimensions of wellness - physical, mental, emotional, and spiritual.

Psychological Aspect: Ageing also has profound psychological implications, impacting one's sense of identity, purpose, and well-being. As individuals navigate the later stages of life, they may grapple with existential questions, loss, and transitions. However, Ageing also offers opportunities for personal growth, self-reflection, and fulfillment as they draw upon their life experiences and wisdom to find meaning and purpose in their lives. Purpose is the driving force to live a life full of zest.

Social Aspect: Finally, Ageing is deeply intertwined with social dynamics and relationships, shaping one's sense of belonging, support, and connectivity. As older adults retire from work and experience changes in social roles and networks, they may face challenges related to loneliness, isolation, and social exclusion. However, Ageing also presents opportunities for building new connections, engAgeing in meaningful activities, and contributing to the community, fostering a sense of purpose and belonging in later life.

The Potential for Growth, Fulfillment, and Transformation in Later Life:

Despite the myths and misconceptions that surround Ageing, the later years of life hold immense potential for growth, fulfillment, and transformation. As individuals embrace the opportunities and challenges of Ageing, they can cultivate resilience, wisdom, and a deeper appreciation for life's joys and blessings. By fostering a positive mindset, nurturing meaningful relationships, and pursuing passions and interests, seniors can thrive in their later years, embodying the true essence of vibrant Ageing.

In conclusion, understanding Ageing requires us to dispel myths, explore realities, and embrace the multidimensional nature of this profound journey. By recognizing the biological, psychological, and social aspects of Ageing, we can gain a deeper appreciation for its complexities and opportunities. Ultimately, Ageing is not a time of decline, but rather a time of growth, fulfillment, and transformation – a journey that has the power to enrich our lives and expand our horizons in ways we never imagined.

"In the end, it's not the years in your life that count. It's the life in your years." - Abraham Lincoln

"True wellness in the golden years isn't just about adding years to life, but about adding life to years."

3

Wellness: The Greatest Asset

Wellness is of paramount importance for all of us. Being proactive to maintain wellness is preserving and enhancing the greatest asset we have: the gift of LIFE.

Holistic wellness for vibrant Ageing encapsulates a comprehensive approach to well-being that nurtures the mind, body, and spirit as individuals advance in age. It involves embracing practices that promote physical health, such as regular exercise, nutritious eating habits, and adequate sleep, while also prioritizing mental and emotional wellness through activities like meditation, mindfulness, and lifelong learning. Additionally, holistic wellness for vibrant Ageing encompasses social connections, fostering meaningful relationships and a sense of belonging within communities. By integrating these elements, individuals can cultivate a sense of vitality, purpose, and fulfillment as they journey through the various stages of Ageing, enabling them to thrive and live their lives to the fullest.

Significance of Holistic Wellness for Seniors:

Here's why holistic wellness holds such significance for seniors:

Quality of Life: Wellness directly impacts the overall quality of life for seniors. By prioritizing physical activity, proper nutrition, mental stimulation, and emotional well-being, seniors can enhance their vitality, mobility, and independence. A focus on wellness enables seniors to be independent and maintain a sense of purpose and fulfillment.

Disease Prevention and Management: Proactive wellness practices play a crucial role in preventing and manAgeing chronic diseases commonly associated with Ageing, such as heart disease, diabetes, osteoporosis, and arthritis. By maintaining a healthy lifestyle and practicing self-care, seniors can reduce their risk of developing these conditions and better manage existing health concerns, thus minimizing the impact on their daily lives.

Mental and Cognitive Health: Wellness initiatives that promote mental and cognitive health are essential for seniors' overall well-being. EngAgeing in activities that stimulate the mind, such as reading, puzzles, and social interaction, can help preserve cognitive function and reduce the risk of cognitive decline and dementia. Additionally, prioritizing emotional wellness through stress management and social support enhances mental resilience and emotional stability.

Social Connection and Support: Wellness extends beyond individual health practices to encompass social connection and support networks. Maintaining meaningful relationships and participating in social activities fosters a sense of belonging and reduces feelings of loneliness and isolation, which are common concerns among seniors. Social interaction also promotes mental stimulation and emotional well-being.

Longevity and Ageing Gracefully: By adopting healthy lifestyle habits and embracing holistic wellness practices, seniors can enhance their longevity and maintain their independence, vitality, and resilience as they navigate the Ageing process.

In conclusion, holistic wellness for seniors encompasses a multidimensional approach to well-being – addressing the interconnected aspects of physical, mental, emotional, and spiritual health. By proactively prioritizing self-care, engAgeing in activities that promote vitality and fulfillment, and seeking support when needed, seniors can embrace the golden years with vitality, purpose, and a profound sense of well-being.

Common Challenges and Opportunities:

As seniors embark on their wellness journey, they encounter a variety of challenges and opportunities that shape their path towards optimal health and well-being.

Understanding these common challenges and opportunities is essential for developing effective strategies to overcome obstacles and capitalize on strengths. Here, we explore some of the most prevalent challenges and opportunities seniors face:

Common Challenges of Seniors:

Physical Limitations: Seniors often contend with age-related physical limitations, such as reduced mobility, strength, and flexibility. These limitations can hinder participation in physical activities and daily tasks, impacting overall well-being and confidence.

Chronic Health Conditions: Many seniors grapple with chronic health conditions, such as arthritis, hypertension, and heart disease. ManAgeing these conditions requires ongoing medical care, lifestyle modifications, and adherence to treatment plans.

Isolation and Loneliness: Social isolation and loneliness are significant concerns among seniors, particularly those living alone or experiencing limited social interaction. Feelings of isolation can lead to depression, anxiety, and decreased quality of life.

Financial Constraints: Limited financial resources can pose challenges for seniors seeking access to healthcare, healthy food options, and wellness programs. Financial constraints may also impact seniors' ability to engage in recreational activities or pursue hobbies.

Opportunities for Seniors:

Community Support: Seniors have the opportunity to leverage community resources and support networks to address challenges and enhance their well-being. Community centers, senior centers, and local organizations offer a variety of programs and services tailored to seniors' needs. Registering themselves with the nearest local organization enables them to get support in times of emergency situations also.

Technology and Innovation: Advancements in technology present opportunities for seniors to improve their health and well-being. From telecommunications for consultation and wearable fitness devices (e.g., CGM continuous glucose monitoring, FITBIT to be aware of the heart rate) to online social networks and virtual fitness classes, technology offers convenient and accessible solutions for seniors seeking to enhance their wellness. The government has created online facilities for senior citizens for banking services, tax filing, and health services from the comfort of home.

Lifelong Learning: Lifelong learning opportunities abound for seniors interested in expanding their knowledge and skills. Whether through formal education programs, online courses, or community workshops, seniors have the chance to pursue intellectual interests and engage in stimulating activities. It empowers them to take proactive measures to address the challenges.

By addressing these challenges and seizing opportunities, seniors can embark on a wellness journey that enhances their overall well-being and enables them to live fulfilling and vibrant lives.

Self-Discovery and Personal Growth:

Ageing presents opportunities for self-discovery and personal growth. Seniors can embrace new hobbies, explore creative pursuits, and reflect on their life experiences, fostering a sense of fulfillment and purpose in their later years. By navigating these challenges and seizing opportunities, seniors can embark on a wellness journey characterized by resilience, empowerment, and fulfillment. By embracing support networks, leverAgeing technology, pursuing lifelong learning, and embracing personal growth, seniors can overcome obstacles and thrive in their golden years. By learning new strategies to tackle challenges or obstacles in day-to-day life, they get an opportunity to enhance their problem-solving ability and thus secretly get a boost in their cognition and confidence.

Integrating Mind, Body, and Spirit in the Pursuit of Wellness:

True wellness goes beyond physical health; it encompasses the harmony of mind, body, and spirit. By nurturing each aspect – mental, physical, and spiritual – seniors can achieve a profound sense of vitality, purpose, and fulfillment in their lives.

Mind: Our subconscious mind is a powerful force that influences our thoughts, emotions, and behaviors. Seniors can enhance mental well-being by practicing mindfulness, saying aloud personalized affirmations, engAgeing in cognitive exercises, and fostering positive thinking patterns. Activities such as meditation, journaling, and visualization techniques can promote mental clarity, emotional resilience, and a sense of inner peace. By cultivating a healthy mindset and manAgeing stress effectively, seniors can harness the power of their minds to navigate life's challenges with grace and resilience. Attitude is everything.

Body: The body is a temple that requires care, nourishment, and movement to thrive. Seniors can promote physical wellness by adopting a balanced diet, staying active, and prioritizing rest and relaxation. Regular exercise, such as walking, yoga, or strength training, can improve strength, flexibility, and cardiovascular health, while also boosting mood and energy levels. Additionally, adequate sleep, hydration, and preventive healthcare measures are essential for maintaining optimal physical health and vitality in later life.

Spirit: The spirit encompasses the essence of our being – our values, beliefs, and sense of purpose in life. Seniors can nurture their spiritual well-being by connecting with nature, engAgeing in meaningful activities, and exploring their sense of purpose and meaning. Practices such as prayer, meditation, or spending time in quiet reflection can deepen one's connection to oneself, others, and the universe at large. By aligning with their innermost values and aspirations, seniors can cultivate a profound sense of fulfillment, contentment, and inner peace.

Integration: Integrating mind, body, and spirit in the pursuit of wellness involves recognizing the interconnectivity of these elements and nurturing them holistically. Seniors can achieve this integration by engAgeing in practices that nourish each aspect of their being – from physical exercise and healthy nutrition to mindfulness and spiritual exploration. By honoring the mind-body-spirit connection, seniors can unlock the full potential of their well-being and experience a profound sense of vitality, purpose, and wholeness in their lives.

While enjoying a morning walk, one can listen to nature's sounds like birds chirping, the sound of flowing water, or the rustling of leaves. Green leaves and colorful butterflies on the bed of flowers are a refreshing treat to the eyes. The soft touch of grass experienced by the feet sole is cool and soothing. The feel of a cool breeze or warmth of the rising sun while meditating in the garden integrates mind, body, and soul.

Meditation:

Meditation, with its quiet strength, serves as the conduit through which mind, body, and spirit unite in perfect harmony. As we close our eyes and delve into the depths of our consciousness, we invite a profound connection between our thoughts, physical sensations, and innermost essence. With each breath, we cultivate awareness, nurturing a sense of balance that transcends the boundaries of our being. In this sacred space, tensions dissolve, clarity emerges, and the whispers of our soul resonate with the rhythm of the universe. Through meditation, we embrace the intricate interplay of our existence, fostering a profound sense of wholeness and serenity that radiates from within.

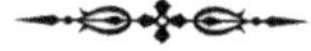

4

OPTIMIZING PHYSICAL HEALTH FOR VIBRANT AGING

Physical health is indeed crucial for vibrant Ageing, providing the foundation for overall well-being and vitality in later life. As individuals age, the accumulation of molecular and cellular damage over time can lead to a gradual decrease in physical and mental capacity, compromising mobility and functional capacity. However, by prioritizing physical wellness, seniors can maintain independence, vitality, and resilience as they age.

Strategies and practices to optimize physical health include:

Nutrition and Hydration: Seniors should prioritize consuming a balanced and nutritious diet rich in fruits, vegetables, whole grains, lean proteins, and healthy fats. Adequate hydration is also essential to prevent dehydration, which can be a risk due to changes in thirst sensation and kidney function.

Exercise and Movement: Regular exercise is vital for promoting physical health and functional capacity in seniors. Incorporating a variety of activities, including aerobic exercise, strength training, flexibility exercises, and balance training, can improve cardiovascular fitness, muscle strength, joint flexibility, and balance. Seniors should aim for at least 150 minutes of moderate-intensity aerobic activity per week, along with muscle-strengthening exercises on two or more days per week.

Preventive Healthcare: Regular check-ups, screenings, and vaccinations are important components of preventive healthcare for seniors. Working closely with healthcare providers to develop personalized preventive healthcare plans based on individual risk factors and health goals is essential.

Lifestyle Choices: Healthy lifestyle choices such as avoiding smoking, limiting alcohol consumption, maintaining a healthy weight, prioritizing sleep, manAgeing stress effectively, and practicing good hygiene and safety habits can significantly impact physical health and well-being in seniors.

Incorporating Physical Activity into Daily Life: Seniors should be encouraged to incorporate physical activity into their daily routines through simple activities such as walking, gardening, household chores, and dancing. Making physical activity a regular part of their lifestyle helps maintain good health over the long term.

In conclusion, optimizing physical health is essential for vibrant Ageing and well-being in seniors. By prioritizing regular exercise, nutritious eating, preventive healthcare, and healthy lifestyle choices, seniors can maintain their physical vitality, independence, and quality of life as they age. Through proactive self-care and a commitment to physical wellness, seniors can embrace the journey of Ageing with strength, resilience, and vitality. These aspects will be explored in detail in the following chapters.

4.1 NOURISHING YOUR BODY

"Nutrition is not just about eating; it's about nourishing your body, mind, and spirit. For seniors, it's the foundation upon which vitality, longevity, and well-being are built."

Nutrition Essentials for vibrant ageing

Nutrition plays a critical role in vibrant Ageing because it directly impacts overall health, vitality, and quality of life as we grow older.

आहारशुद्धौ सत्वशुद्धिः सत्वशुद्धौ ध्रुवा स्मृतिः।स्मृतिलम्भे सर्वग्रंथीनां विप्रमोक्षः॥

Translation: "When diet is pure, the mind is pure; when the mind is pure, memory becomes firm; and when memory is firm, all bonds are loosened."

In this chapter, we delve into the essential components of a healthy diet for vibrant ageing, providing practical guidance and insights to support optimal nutrition and well-being.

Let us understand why nutrition is more important for vibrant Ageing:

1. Supports Physical Health: Proper nutrition provides the essential nutrients needed to support physical health and function. Nutrient-dense foods supply vitamins, minerals, antioxidants, and macro nutrients that support organ function, immune function, tissue repair, and energy production. A well-balanced diet helps maintain muscle mass, bone density, cardiovascular health, immunity and overall vitality, allowing seniors to remain active, independent, and resilient as they age.

2. Promotes Cognitive Function: Certain nutrients are essential for brain health and cognitive function. Omega-3 fatty acids, antioxidants, and vitamins B6, B12, and folate play key roles in supporting memory, concentration, and overall brain health. By consuming a diet rich in these nutrients, seniors can support cognitive function, reduce the risk of cognitive decline, and maintain mental clarity and acuity as they age. Don't forget to include a salad bowl of Dark green leaf salad with steamed broccoli and a dressing of olive oil and sunflower seeds.

3. Aids in Disease Prevention: Proper nutrition can help prevent or manage chronic diseases that become more prevalent with age, such as heart disease, diabetes, osteoporosis, and certain cancers. Besides nourishment it also boosts your immunity to safeguard against common infections.

A diet rich in fruits, vegetables, whole grains, lean proteins, and healthy fats provides the nutrients and antioxidants needed to boost immunity, reduce inflammation, lower cholesterol levels, regulate blood sugar, and support overall health. By adopting a healthy eating pattern, seniors can reduce their risk of developing chronic diseases and improve their overall quality of life.

1. Harmonizes Digestive Health: As we age, digestive health becomes increasingly important for nutrient absorption, immune function, and overall well-being. A diet high in fiber from fruits, vegetables, whole grains, and legumes promotes digestive regularity, prevents constipation, and supports a healthy gut micro-biome. Adequate hydration and consumption of pro-biotic-rich foods further support digestive health, reducing the risk of gastrointestinal issues and promoting overall vitality.

2. Boosts Energy and Vitality: Proper nutrition provides the energy and nutrients needed to fuel daily activities and maintain vitality throughout the ageing process. Nutrient-rich foods supply carbohydrates for energy, protein for muscle repair and maintenance, and healthy fats for sustained energy and satiety. By consuming a balanced diet that meets their individual energy needs, seniors can maintain energy levels, prevent fatigue, and enjoy an active and vibrant lifestyle.

3. Supports Skin and Bone Health: Nutrients such as vitamins C, E, and A, along with minerals like zinc and calcium, are essential for skin and bone health. A diet rich in fruits, vegetables, lean proteins, and dairy products provides the

nutrients needed to support collagen production, protect against oxidative damage, and maintain bone density and strength. By prioritizing these nutrients, seniors can support skin elasticity, hydration, and overall appearance, as well as reduce the risk of osteoporosis and fractures.

In summary, nutrition is more important for vibrant Ageing because it directly impacts physical health, cognitive function, disease prevention, digestive health, energy levels, and overall vitality. By prioritizing nutrient-rich foods and adopting healthy eating habits, seniors can support their well-being, enhance their quality of life, and age vibrantly with grace and resilience.

MIND MAP

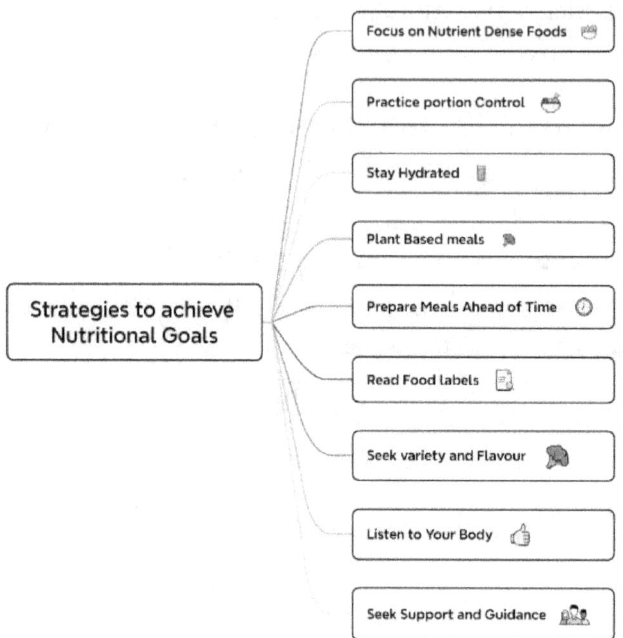

Understanding Senior Nutritional Needs

As we age, our nutritional needs evolve, requiring adjustments to dietary habits to ensure adequate nutrient intake. Changes in metabolism, appetite, digestion, and nutrient absorption may occur, making it imperative to prioritize nutrient-dense foods that support optimal health and vitality. In this chapter, we'll explore in detail how to meet these nutritional criteria through a balanced and varied diet, along with practical tips for implementation.

1. Focus on Nutrient-Dense Foods:

Nutrient-dense foods are rich in essential nutrients while being relatively low in calories. They provide vitamins, minerals, antioxidants, and phytonutrients that are crucial for supporting health and well-being. Examples of nutrient-dense foods include fruits, vegetables, lean proteins, whole grains, nuts, seeds, and legumes. Incorporating a variety of these foods into your diet ensures that you meet your body's nutritional needs without excess calories or unhealthy additives.

2. Prioritize Protein-Rich Foods:

Protein is essential for maintaining muscle mass, bone health, and overall strength, particularly as we age. Older adults absorb protein less effectively and require 0.54 grams of protein per pound of body weight per day. If you weigh 68 kilograms (150 pounds), you need to eat 81 grams of protein (J. Brody et al.).

Seniors should aim to include protein-rich foods in each meal, such as lean meats, poultry, fish, eggs, dairy products, tofu, legumes, pulses, nuts, and seeds. Incorporating a variety of protein sources ensures that you receive all essential amino acids necessary for tissue repair and maintenance.

The most effective proteins as we age are those that are rich in the amino acid leucine. Leucine is one of the nine essential amino acids (building blocks of proteins) that we need to obtain through our diet. Plan a portion of proteins in each meal. Choose proteins that are best suitable for digestion, seasonal, locally available, and in the most natural digestible form. Too much heat processing of protein-rich foods should be avoided. The natural process of soaking and sprouting of pulses and nuts complements digestion and better availability of nutrients for assimilation.

3. Emphasize Plant-Based Foods:

Plant-based foods are rich in fiber, vitamins, minerals, and antioxidants that support overall health and longevity. Aim to fill half of your plate with fruits and vegetables at each meal, choosing a variety of colors and types to maximize nutrient intake. Include whole grains such as brown rice, quinoa, oats, and whole wheat bread, along with legumes such as beans, lentils, and chickpeas, to provide fiber, protein, and essential nutrients.

4. Incorporate Healthy Fats:

Healthy fats are essential for heart health, brain function, and inflammation control. Fats are a major source of energy and they're necessary for building the myelin sheath around neurons and maintaining strong and healthy cells. Include sources of unsaturated fats such as olive oil, avocados, nuts, seeds, and fatty fish (e.g., salmon, mackerel, sardines) in your diet regularly. Limit sources of saturated and trans fats found in processed and fried foods, as well as baked goods and high-fat dairy products, to reduce the risk of heart disease and other chronic conditions.

Diets high in soluble fibers are good because the fiber binds to the LDL molecules, the bad cholesterol, in the digestive system and drags them out of the body before they get into circulation. Whole grains, sprouted pulses, salads, vegetables, fruits, chia seeds, flax seeds, hemp seeds, and coconut chutney are good sources of fiber. Diets high in Omega-3 fatty acids, as found in seeds (especially chia, flax, hemp), walnuts, and olive and canola oil, also lower LDL and reduce the risk of heart disease by 7 percent (Chowdhury et al.).

5. Stay Hydrated:

Aristotle wrote that "living beings are moist and warm... however old age is dry and cold." The classical Greek physician Galen of Pergamon added that "Ageing is associated with a decline in innate heat and body water." Galen further lamented that dehydration is difficult to diagnose. It is most problematic among children and adults over seventy.

Hydration is essential for cellular and brain health. Dehydration is a medical condition; it is not just thirst. Thirst is just a symptom of dehydration. Dehydration is deadly. It's the eighth leading cause of death among adults over seventy (C. Troeger et al.). It is also linked to the formation of kidney stones. Common causes are too much heat or exercise (because you lose salts through your sweat), higher altitudes, and illness. Alcohol is also a culprit: It turns off hormones that help us absorb water so we lose more fluids than normal.

Individuals at the greatest risk for dehydration include people with fever or infections, impaired cognitive status, or impaired renal function, and those who are on diuretic medications. Dehydration occurs from an imbalance of water, salt, and electrolytes in the blood. Electrolytes include sodium, chloride, potassium, and magnesium. Rehydrating doesn't mean simply drinking more water because when you are dehydrated, the body can't retain the water you drink, and water alone does not replace the depleted salts and electrolytes.

Rehydration requires drinking oral rehydration salts (ORS) solutions. An ORS is a mixture of salt and electrolytes; it is absorbed in the small intestine and replaces the water and electrolytes lost in dehydration.

For maintaining hydration, aim to drink plenty of water throughout the day, and include hydrating foods such as fruits, vegetables, soups, and herbal teas in your diet. Pay attention to thirst cues and increase fluid intake during hot weather or periods of increased physical activity to prevent dehydration and support optimal bodily functions.

Meet Calcium and Vitamin D Needs:

Calcium and vitamin D are crucial for maintaining bone health and preventing osteoporosis. Include calcium-rich foods such as dairy products, fortified plant-based milks, leafy green vegetables (e.g., kale, collard greens, broccoli), and fortified foods (e.g., tofu, orange juice) in your diet regularly. Aim for at least 1,200 milligrams of calcium per day for women over 50 and men over 70. Additionally, get adequate sunlight exposure or consider vitamin D supplementation to support vitamin D levels and calcium absorption.

Focus on Whole Foods:

Prioritize whole, minimally processed foods over highly processed and refined options. Whole foods are higher in nutrients and fiber and lower in added sugars, sodium, and unhealthy fats. Choose whole grains such as brown rice, quinoa, Jawar, barley, and millets over refined grains, and opt for fresh fruits and vegetables instead of canned varieties with added sugars or preservatives. Cooking meals from scratch using whole ingredients allows you to control the quality and nutritional content of your meals.

Practice Portion Control:

Pay attention to portion sizes to avoid overeating and maintain a healthy weight. Use smaller plates and bowls, and be mindful of serving sizes when dining out or preparing meals at home. Aim to fill half of your plate with fruits and vegetables, one-quarter with protein, and one-quarter with whole grains or starchy vegetables to create balanced and satisfying meals. Avoid eating until you're overly full and listen to your body's hunger and fullness cues to prevent overconsumption.

Summary of healthy eating habits and meal planning strategies to achieve nutritional goals:

1. Prioritize Nutrient-Rich Foods:

- Fill your plate with a variety of colorful fruits and vegetables, aiming for at least five servings per day.

- Choose whole grains such as brown rice, quinoa, oats, and whole wheat bread over refined grains.

- Incorporate protein from varied sources such as poultry, fish, beans, lentils, tofu, sprouted grains, and nuts.

- Include healthy fats from sources like avocados, nuts, seeds, and olive oil.

2. Practice Portion Control:

- Pay attention to portion sizes to avoid overeating. Use measuring cups, spoons, or visual cues to gauge serving sizes.

- Opt for smaller plates and bowls to help control portion sizes and prevent overeating.

- Be mindful of portion distortion when dining out, as restaurant servings are often larger than necessary.

3. Stay Hydrated:

- Drink plenty of water throughout the day to stay hydrated and support optimal bodily functions.

- Limit consumption of sugary beverages, caffeinated drinks, and alcohol, which can contribute to dehydration.

4. Plan Balanced Meals:

- Build meals around a combination of protein, whole grains, healthy fats, fiber, and plenty of fruits and vegetables.

- Aim for a balance of macronutrients (carbohydrates, protein, and fat) to support energy levels and overall health.

- Incorporate a variety of textures, flavors, and colors to make meals more appealing and satisfying.

5. Prepare Meals Ahead of Time:

- Set aside time for meal prep to make healthy eating more convenient and accessible.

- Batch cook staples such as grains, proteins, and vegetables to use in multiple meals throughout the week.

6. Read Food Labels:

- Pay attention to nutrition labels when purchasing packaged foods to make informed choices about nutrient content and portion sizes.

- Look for products with minimal added sugars, sodium, preservatives, and unhealthy fats.

7. Seek Variety and Flavor:

- Experiment with new foods, flavors, and recipes to keep meals interesting and enjoyable.

- Incorporate a variety of herbs, spices, and seasonings to enhance the taste of meals without relying on excessive salt or sugar.

8. Listen to Your Body:

- Eat mindfully, paying attention to hunger and fullness cues to avoid overeating.

- Practice mindful eating by savoring each bite, chewing slowly, and appreciating the flavors and textures of your food.

9. Seek Support and Guidance:

- Consult with a registered dietitian or nutritionist for personalized meal planning advice and dietary recommendations.

- Join community cooking classes, support groups, or wellness programs to connect with others and share healthy eating tips and recipes.

MIND MAP

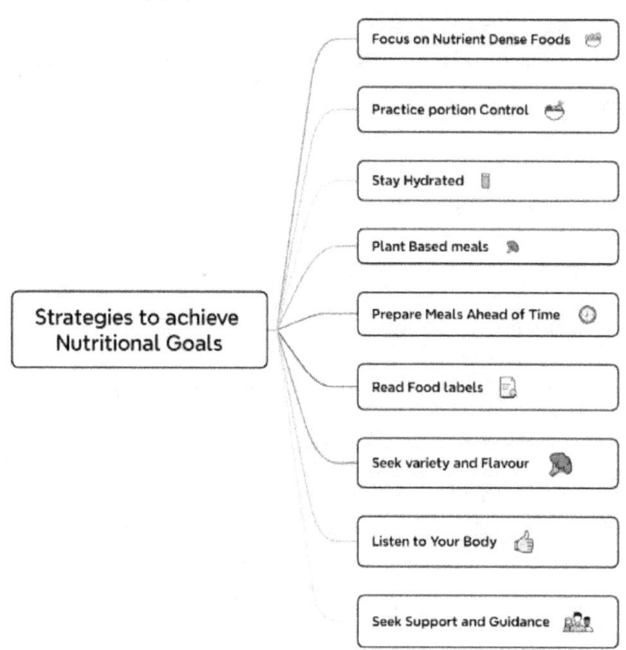

ManAgeing Dietary Challenges and Restrictions

Seniors may face various dietary challenges and restrictions due to health conditions, allergies, intolerance, or personal preferences. Effectively manAgeing these challenges is essential for maintaining optimal health and well-being. Here's a guide to help seniors navigate common dietary challenges and restrictions:

1. Food Allergies and Intolerance:

- Identify and avoid foods that trigger allergic reactions or intolerance, such as dairy, gluten, nuts, and spices.

- Read food labels carefully to check for potential allergens and hidden ingredients.

- Experiment with alternative ingredients and substitutions to accommodate dietary restrictions while still enjoying flavorful meals. For example, if an individual becomes intolerant to milk and milk products, then alternative protein and calcium substitutes can be planned, such as oat milk, coconut milk, or almond milk.

2. Chronic Health Conditions:

- Seniors with chronic health conditions such as diabetes, hypertension, heart disease, or kidney disease may need to follow specific dietary guidelines.

- Work closely with healthcare providers and registered dietitians to develop personalized meal plans that address individual health needs and goals.

- Monitor blood sugar levels, blood pressure, cholesterol levels, and other relevant health markers regularly to assess the impact of dietary changes.

3. Digestive Issues:

- Seniors experiencing digestive issues such as acid reflux, irritable bowel syndrome (IBS), or constipation may benefit from dietary modifications.

- Focus on easily digestible foods such as cooked vegetables, easy-to-digest proteins, whole grains, and low-fat dairy products.

- Limit intake of spicy, fatty, or processed foods that may exacerbate digestive symptoms.

- Include properly cooked, soaked, or roasted powdered food grains that are easy to chew and digest.

4. Dental Problems:

- Seniors with dental problems such as missing teeth, gum disease, or difficulty chewing may struggle to eat certain foods.

- Opt for soft, easily chewable foods such as mashed vegetables, smoothies, soups, yogurt, and cooked grains.

- Use kitchen tools such as blenders, food processors, or immersion blenders to puree or blend foods for easier consumption.

5. Medication Interactions:

- Some medications may interact with certain foods or nutrients, affecting absorption, metabolism, or effectiveness.

- Consult with healthcare providers or pharmacists to understand potential interactions and make appropriate dietary adjustments if necessary.

- Take medications as directed, with or without food, according to healthcare provider recommendations.

6. Social and Cultural Factors:

- Consider social and cultural preferences, traditions, and dietary practices when planning meals and making food choices.

- Find ways to incorporate familiar foods and flavors from cultural backgrounds while still meeting nutritional needs and dietary goals.

- Enjoy meals with family, friends, or community members as a way to share cultural traditions and strengthen social connections.

7. Psychological and Emotional Factors:

- Emotional factors such as stress, depression, anxiety, or loneliness can impact appetite and eating habits.

- Practice self-care strategies such as stress management, relaxation techniques, and engAgeing in enjoyable activities to support emotional well-being.

- Seek support from healthcare professionals, counselors, or support groups if psychological factors are affecting dietary habits.

8. Stay Informed and Educated:

 - Stay informed about dietary recommendations, nutrition trends, and emerging research related to specific health conditions or dietary restrictions.

- Attend educational workshops, seminars, or webinars to learn more about manAgeing dietary challenges and optimizing nutrition in later life.

Ultimately, by addressing dietary challenges and restrictions proactively and seeking personalized guidance when needed, seniors can take control of their diet and nutrition, leading to improved health outcomes and a higher quality of life in their golden years.

A prayer before consuming food:

"Our mindset and emotional state matter a lot while consuming food. Mindful eating in a calm and peaceful environment fulfills the purpose of nourishing and rejuvenating to age vibrantly."

In Hindu tradition, there is a beautiful prayer which is said before eating food.

ॐ सह नाववतु। सह नौ भुनक्तु। सह वीर्यं करवावहै। तेजस्वि नावधीतमस्तु मा विद्विषावहै। ॐ शान्तिः शान्तिः शान्तिः॥

This Sanskrit prayer translates to:

"May we together be protected, May we together be nourished, May we work together with great energy, May our study be enlightening, May there be no hatred between us, Om peace, peace, peace."

4.2 STAYING ACTIVE AND FIT

"Fitness is not about being better than someone else; it's about being better than you used to be." - Unknown

"Take care of your body. It's the only place you have to live."
- Jim Rohn

The Benefits of Physical Activity for Seniors

Being fit and healthy is the foundation not only of physical wellness but also of emotional and mental wellness.

The joy of enjoying exuberant health empowers us to defy Ageing. Just imagine and visualize living an extra decade of glorious life

To enjoy that ultra-healthy life

As Robin Sharma beautifully said:

*Healthset is all about dialing in your physical dimension so
your brain is operating at its highest level of cognition and
so your energy is igniting and so your stress is dissolving and
so your joy is expanding.*

Physical activity is a cornerstone of Ageing with grace, offering a multitude of benefits that contribute to overall health, vitality, and quality of life. In this chapter, we explore the numerous advantages of staying active and fit as we age, highlighting the importance of incorporating regular exercise into daily life.

1. Enhanced Physical Health:

Regular physical activity lubricates the entire body and creates momentum in all physiological systems. With an increased heart rate, blood circulates at a faster rate, simultaneously nourishing and supplying nutrients to vital organs and cells. Exercise supports cardiovascular health, improving heart function, lowering blood pressure, and reducing the risk of heart disease, stroke, and diabetes. It also facilitates the elimination of toxins from the body through breath, sweat, and excretion.

Breathing deeply increases lung capacity, enabling more oxygen to be inhaled, which is essential for physiological functioning and metabolism. Elevated metabolism fuels the body's fat-burning engine, enabling more efficient burning of excess fat. Exercise helps maintain strength, flexibility, and endurance, reducing the risk of falls, fractures, and other injuries. Weight-bearing activities such as walking, yoga, or strength training help maintain bone density and prevent osteoporosis.

2. Improved Mental Health:

Exercising in the morning generates an alchemy in your brain based on neurophysiology, electrifying momentum in your body and energizing and setting your neurons into the arena of focus and memorization.

Morning exercise helps in reducing the stress and fear hormone, cortisol, which stunts growth, immunity, and well-being. Scientific data confirms that cortisol levels are highest in the morning. Just a 30-minute routine of morning exercise implemented consistently significantly lowers cortisol.

Science has also presented a vital link between physical fitness and cognitive ability. Sweating from a powerful workout releases BDNF (brain-derived neurotrophic factor), which elevates brain energy. BDNF repairs brain cells damaged by stress, accelerates the formation of neural connections, and promotes neurogenesis. This offsets the risk of dementia and Alzheimer's disease in later life.

Exercise also leads to the release of dopamine, the neurotransmitter of drive and motivation, along with elevating serotonin levels, boosting happiness quotient, and keeping you purposeful. Dopamine boosts norepinephrine, improving attention and leaving you feeling serene. Furthermore, exercise regulates the amygdala in the limbic system, preparing you to respond to challenges in a more rational and thoughtful manner.

In summary, physical activity and exercise boost mood, concentration, memory, reduce symptoms of depression and anxiety, and enhance overall mental well-being in seniors.

3. Enhanced Quality of Life:

Staying active allows seniors to maintain independence, mobility, and functional ability, enabling them to engage in daily activities and hobbies with ease. Regular exercise fosters social connections and opportunities for interaction, reducing feelings of loneliness and isolation commonly experienced by seniors. Physical activity provides a sense of purpose and fulfillment, promoting a higher quality of life and greater overall satisfaction with health and well-being.

4. Longevity and Healthy Ageing:

Research has shown that regular exercise is associated with increased longevity and a lower risk of premature death in older adults. By promoting overall health and well-being, physical activity supports healthy Ageing, allowing seniors to enjoy a longer, more active, and independent lifestyle. Exercise helps manage chronic health conditions and age-related ailments, allowing seniors to maintain a higher quality of life and age gracefully.

In summary, the benefits of physical activity for seniors are vast and multifaceted, encompassing improvements in physical health, mental well-being, quality of life, and longevity. By incorporating regular exercise into your daily routine, you can enhance your overall health, vitality, and happiness, enabling you to live life to the fullest in your golden years.

Tailoring Exercise to Your Needs and Abilities:

Before starting any exercise regimen, seniors should consult with their healthcare provider to assess their current health status and receive personalized recommendations. Seniors should select activities that align with their interests, physical abilities, and health goals. This could range from low-impact exercises like walking or swimming to more structured activities such as tai chi or yoga.

Gradual Progression:

It's essential for seniors to start slowly and gradually increase the intensity and duration of their workouts to prevent injuries and accommodate their fitness level.

Incorporating Strength Training:

Strength training exercises, using resistance bands or light weights, are crucial for maintaining muscle mass and bone density, both of which decline with age.

Flexibility and Balance Exercises:

Stretching and balance exercises are vital for improving flexibility, reducing the risk of falls, and enhancing overall mobility.

Listening to Your Body:

Seniors should pay attention to their bodies and adjust their exercise routines accordingly. It's essential to recognize signs of fatigue or discomfort and modify activities as needed.

Here is a list of a few simple physical exercises that can be chosen according to individual suitability and incorporated into your daily fitness routine after discussing with a healthcare expert.

1. Walking: Walking is a low-impact exercise that provides cardiovascular benefits and strengthens muscles. Aim for at least 30 minutes of brisk walking most days of the week. Consider walking outdoors in nature for added mental health benefits.

2. Strength Training with Resistance Bands: Resistance bands offer a gentle yet effective way to build muscle strength and endurance. Perform exercises such as bicep curls, shoulder presses, leg lifts, and seated rows using resistance bands. Start with light resistance and gradually increase as you build strength.

3. Chair Yoga: Chair yoga is a gentle form of yoga that can be done while seated or using a chair for support. It improves flexibility, balance, and relaxation. Try simple chair yoga poses such as seated twists, gentle stretches, and deep breathing exercises to promote mobility and reduce stress.

4. Balance Exercises: Improving balance is crucial for preventing falls and maintaining independence. Practice standing on one leg while holding onto a sturdy chair or countertop for support. Gradually progress to standing on one leg without support, or try balancing exercises such as heel-to-toe walking or standing yoga poses.

5. Tai Chi: Tai Chi is a slow, flowing martial art that promotes balance, flexibility, and relaxation. It involves gentle, rhythmic movements combined with deep breathing and mindfulness. Join a Tai Chi class designed for older adults or follow along with instructional videos online to reap the benefits of this ancient practice.

6. Water Aerobics: Water aerobics is a low-impact exercise performed in water that provides resistance and buoyancy. It's gentle on the joints while still offering a cardiovascular workout and muscle-strengthening benefits. Look for water aerobics classes at local pools or try exercises such as water walking, leg lifts, and arm circles in a shallow pool.

7. Flexibility Exercises: Stretching exercises help maintain flexibility and range of motion in joints, reducing the risk of injury and improving overall mobility. Perform gentle stretches for major muscle groups, focusing on areas such as the neck, shoulders, back, hips, and legs. Hold each stretch for 15-30 seconds and repeat several times.

8. Dance: Dancing is a fun and enjoyable way to stay active while improving cardiovascular health, coordination, and mood. Put on some music and dance around your living room, or join a dance class tailored for older adults. Choose dance styles such as ballroom, line dancing, or salsa that are low-impact and easy on the joints.

Remember to consult with a healthcare professional before starting any new exercise program, especially if you have pre-existing health conditions or concerns. Start slowly, listen to your body, and gradually increase intensity and duration as your fitness level improves. Enjoy the process of staying active and reaping the numerous physical and mental health benefits that exercise provides!

In conclusion, by embracing regular physical activity and tailoring exercise routines to individual needs and abilities, older adults can enjoy numerous benefits of vibrant Ageing, including improved physical and mental well-being, social engagement, and independence. With proper guidance and commitment, seniors can maintain an active lifestyle well into their golden years.

Overcoming Barriers to Exercise and Maintaining Motivation:

Identifying Barriers: The first step in overcoming barriers to exercise is to identify them. Common barriers for seniors may include physical limitations, lack of motivation, time constraints, fear of injury, or simply feeling too tired.

Setting Realistic Goals: Seniors should set realistic and achievable goals based on their abilities and circumstances. Breaking down larger goals into smaller, manageable tasks can make them feel more attainable. Keeping in mind that small actions today will lay stepping stones for more actions and momentum tomorrow. So practicing patience and perseverance is the key to vibrant Ageing.

Finding Enjoyable Activities: EngAgeing in activities that are enjoyable and interesting can help maintain motivation. Whether it's dancing, gardening, yoga, morning club, or joining a walking group, finding activities that seniors genuinely enjoy can make exercise feel less like a chore.

Creating a Supportive Environment: Having a supportive environment can significantly impact motivation. This could involve exercising with a friend or family member, joining group classes, or seeking encouragement from peers who share similar fitness goals. Support from a community with similar interests helps in finding solutions to problem areas. Also, exercising in a group provides an opportunity for social connection and a greater purpose for community welfare. It alleviates the problem of feeling isolated and bored.

Adapting to Physical Limitations: Seniors should work with healthcare professionals or fitness experts to adapt exercises to accommodate any physical limitations or health concerns. There are often modified versions of exercises that can be performed to suit individual needs.

Incorporating Variety: Monotony can be a major deterrent to exercise. Seniors can keep things interesting by incorporating variety into their workouts. This could involve trying different types of exercises, exploring new outdoor activities, or participating in recreational sports.

Utilizing Technology and Resources: Human nature is such that unless we are accountable to someone for regular exercise, we lack motivation in pursuing it consistently. Technology can be a valuable accountability tool for staying motivated and tracking progress. Many smartphones and wearable devices offer fitness apps or trackers that can monitor activity levels and provide feedback. Additionally, there are numerous online resources, such as exercise videos or virtual fitness classes, that seniors can access from the comfort of their homes.

Rewarding Progress: Celebrating small victories and milestones along the way can help maintain motivation. Rewards lead to the release of Dopamine, a happy hormone. Whether it's treating oneself to a favorite meal, purchasing new workout gear, or simply acknowledging progress, rewards can reinforce positive behavior and encourage continued commitment to exercise.

Staying Flexible: It's important for seniors to be flexible and adapt their exercise routines as needed. Life can be unpredictable, and there may be times when sticking to a strict workout schedule is challenging. Being flexible and willing to adjust plans when necessary can help prevent feelings of frustration and maintain long-term motivation.

By addressing barriers to exercise and implementing strategies to maintain motivation, seniors can overcome obstacles and continue to enjoy the numerous benefits of staying active and fit well. Being fit is the secret to Ageing vibrantly.

4.3 MINDFUL BREATHING

Mindful Breathing is the key to a Healthy life and Vibrant Ageing. Your breath is your power source. It's an involuntary activity which is the only source of the most important and powerful energy for the body: air loaded with oxygen and prana energy. Breathing is an activity which goes on from external to internal and from internal to external continuously from the time you are born until you breathe your last. When you inhale, you are drawing in many things along with oxygen. When you exhale, you are expelling many toxins, including carbon dioxide. Breathing is normally an involuntary activity which continues even while we are in deep sleep. The rate and depth of breathing are directly related to our emotional and mental state. In an anxious or stressful state, breath is shallow and at a faster rate. Conversely, while the mind is in a calm state or meditative state, breath is deep and longer. If this is done mindfully, your health will be better. Your immune system will be better. It has a positive impact on concentration, memory, and alleviating stress. It enables harmonizing metabolic processes inside our cells. Scientifically, Breathing techniques have been proven to have a therapeutic impact on our mind and body.

Lungs are part of the respiratory system. Lungs are composed of millions of tiny air sacs called alveoli. Alveoli are the functional units of the lungs where gas exchange takes place. Oxygen from inhaled air diffuses into the bloodstream, while carbon dioxide, a waste product, diffuses out of the blood and into the alveoli to be exhaled. At complete rest, the typical adult male exchanges approximately 0.5 L (500 mL; 400 mL for females) of air per breath (tidal volume) at a rate of 12 times per minute, resulting in a minute ventilation rate of about 6 L of air per minute. The volume of air breathed in depends upon lung capacity and heart rate. That means the slower the heart rate, the deeper and longer the breath. The more volume of air we inhale and exhale. Especially with Ageing, the capacity of your lungs to handle more volume of air, and thus purification of blood, reduces. But by systematic conscious practice of various breathing techniques, you can enhance the capacity of your lungs and garner myriad benefits of breathing exercises. The entire process of breathing is regulated by the respiratory system.

There are many techniques of breathing.

1. Deep Belly Breathing (Diaphragmatic Breathing): Deep abdominal breathing is one of the basic techniques, a natural breathing technique like an infant, to be practiced intentionally. Sit or lie down comfortably with your spine straight and shoulders relaxed. Place one hand on your chest and the other on your abdomen. Inhale deeply through your nose, allowing your abdomen to rise as you fill your lungs with air. Exhale slowly and completely through your mouth, feeling your abdomen fall. Repeat for several breaths, focusing on the sensation of deep breathing and the movement of your abdomen.

2. 4-7-8 Breathing Technique: This technique, popularized by Dr. Andrew Weil, involves inhaling for a count of 4, holding the breath

for a count of 7, and exhaling slowly for a count of 8. Sit or lie down in a comfortable position with your eyes closed. Inhale quietly through your nose for a count of 4, then hold your breath for a count of 7. Finally, exhale slowly and completely through your mouth for a count of 8. Repeat the cycle for several rounds, allowing each breath to become slower and more relaxed.

3. Alternate Nostril Breathing (Nadi Shodhana): Sit comfortably with your spine straight and shoulders relaxed. Place your left hand on your left knee with your palm facing upward. Bring your right hand to your nose, using your thumb to close your right nostril and your ring finger to close your left nostril. Start by closing your right nostril and inhaling deeply through your left nostril. Then, close your left nostril and exhale slowly and completely through your right nostril. Inhale through your right nostril, then close it and exhale through your left nostril. Repeat for several rounds, alternating nostrils with each breath.

4. Pursed Lip Breathing: Sit comfortably with your spine straight and shoulders relaxed. Inhale slowly and deeply through your nose. Then, purse your lips as if you're about to blow out a candle and exhale slowly and gently through your mouth. Focus on making your exhale twice as long as your inhale, allowing your breath to be smooth and controlled. Pursed lip breathing can help improve lung function, reduce shortness of breath, and promote relaxation.

5. Progressive Muscle Relaxation with Breathing: Combine deep breathing with progressive muscle relaxation to further enhance relaxation and reduce tension in the body. Start by taking a few deep breaths to calm your mind and body. Then, systematically tense and relax each muscle group in your body, starting from your toes and

working your way up to your head. As you tense each muscle group, inhale deeply, and as you relax, exhale fully. Focus on the sensation of release and relaxation with each exhale.

These breathing techniques can be practiced daily as part of a relaxation routine or whenever you feel stressed, anxious, or in need of calming. They are simple, effective, and can be adapted to suit individual preferences and needs. Incorporating regular breathing exercises into your routine can help promote a sense of calm, balance, and vitality as you age.

Let us briefly understand the benefits of breathing exercises.

- Stress Reduction: Breathing exercises, such as deep breathing or diaphragmatic breathing, reduce the production of stress hormones like cortisol, leading to a calmer and more relaxed state of mind.

- Improved Lung Function: Regular practice of breathing exercises can enhance lung capacity and efficiency, allowing for better oxygen exchange in the body.

- Enhanced Oxygenation: Effective breathing techniques ensure that your body receives an ample supply of oxygen, which is vital for maintaining overall health and providing energy to your cells and organs.

- Improved Focus and Concentration: Conscious and controlled breathing exercises can help increase focus and mental clarity. They can also alleviate symptoms of brain fog and enhance cognitive function.

- Anxiety and Stress Reduction: Breathing exercises reduce anxiety, stress, and symptoms of anxiety disorders. They can help regulate the body's response to stress and promote a sense of calm.

- Pain Management: Deep breathing exercises can help reduce the perception of pain by promoting relaxation and releasing endorphins, the body's natural painkillers.

- Better Sleep: Rhythmic breathing techniques, like the 3-6-3 method, can be used to help you relax before bedtime and improve the quality of your sleep.

- Emotional Regulation: Breathing exercises can help you become more aware of your emotions and respond to them in a controlled and balanced manner. This can be beneficial in managing anger, frustration, or other strong emotions.

- Improved Physical Performance: Athletes often use specific breathing techniques to optimize their performance and increase endurance during physical activities.

- Heart Health: Controlled, deep breathing can reduce blood pressure and promote overall cardiovascular health.

- Immune System Support: Stress reduction through breathing exercises may contribute to a stronger immune system and better overall health.

- Resilience and Coping: Learning to control your breath can be a valuable tool in managing challenging situations, as it can help you stay composed and make more reasoned decisions.

- Mind-Body Connection: Breathing exercises can deepen your awareness of the mind-body connection, promoting a holistic sense of well-being and self-awareness.

Breathe deeply and move boldly; for in the rhythm of your breath and the beat of your heart, you'll find the strength to conquer any challenge.

As you breathe, you're creating space for your best self to emerge. Keep moving, keep breathing, and keep evolving.

5

Cultivating Mental and Emotional Well-Being for Vibrant Aging in Seniors

As seniors embark on the journey of Ageing

Society often thinks of health as something biological and physical: the condition of our bodies

Mental well-being

Before examining what mental well-being is

It is not:

- The absence of mental illness.

- The lack of problems

In fact

So what exactly is this idea of mental well-being?

Mental well-being is how we respond to life's ups and downs. In this simple mental well-being definition lie deeper meaning and implication for our lives. It includes how a person thinks

This important part of who we are has multiple meanings. These traits—which are all actually skills we can practice and develop—are all part of mental well-being:

- Self-acceptance

- Sense of self as part of something greater

- Sense of self as independent rather than dependent on others for identity or happiness

- Knowing and using our unique character strengths

- Accurate perception of reality

- Desire for continued growth

- Thriving in the face of adversity (emotional resilience)

- Having and pursuing interests

- Knowing and remaining true to values

- Maintaining emotionally healthy relationships.

- Optimism (hope—the mindset that things can improve)

- Happiness that comes from within rather than being dependent on external conditions

- Determination

- Action (in contrast to a passive mindset and lifestyle

Examples of Mental Well-being:

Well-being exists in myriad ways. These mental well-being examples are but a handful of ways people can be mentally healthy:

- The man who loses his job and uses his love of learning to take some classes to start a new career path that better matches his passions

- The woman who makes it a point to attend or visit concerts

- The teen athlete who is cut from a team so

- The woman who once experienced a period of homelessness and now gives back by volunteering in the organizations that helped her in the past

- The man who lost his wife in COVID and gets back to life by volunteering to work for an NGO working on Rehabilitation of orphans.

- The human being with anxiety and depression who gets out of bed every single day

Let us look into What is Emotional well-being.

Emotional well-being is the ability to produce positive emotions

One of its foundations is resilience

As you move on on your journey of life

According to the Mental Health Foundation and the CDC: "A positive sense of well-being... enables an individual to be able to function in society and meet the demands of everyday life. Well-being generally includes global judgments of life satisfaction and feelings ranging from depression to joy."

How you deal with your range of emotions is critical.

What's the relationship between emotional well-being and health?

Everything in your life — emotional, social, spiritual, physical, and intellectual — connects in a state of well-being. For example, walking just 10-15 minutes a day gives your brain a boost. That means more energy, awareness, and a healthier outlook on life. Because exercise of any sort balances your dopamine and serotonin levels, it also improves your sleep and reduces stress and anxiety. All of this can make you better equipped to manage your feelings and emotions.

Each area of your well-being has the potential to impact other areas. Many research studies focus on how poor emotional well-being negatively impacts physical health — leading to an increased risk in cancer, heart disease, and respiratory disease. And there is an emerging set of data that is focusing on the effects of positive well-being.

What are some emotional well-being examples?

Strong emotional well-being means you're prepared to face events that may or may not be in your control. When faced with a challenging situation, you might use one of these strategies to bring yourself into a frame of mind that allows you to manage your emotions.

You breathe, ground yourself, and pause.

In a stressful situation, this simple three-step process can help you better control your emotions.

Breathe: When you breathe deeply, you send a message to your brain that helps you calm down and relax.

Ground yourself: Hold a pen. Grab the edge of a desk. Feel the floor under your feet. You return to the present moment and away from your challenging thoughts.

Pause: Wait. Now consider, "What do I really want to say?" When you know the words that will express what you need to communicate, you are in a state of emotional well-being.

You respond instead of react.

To respond is to exercise emotional intelligence. To react is to be emotional. So how do you consistently respond instead of react? Begin by slowing down the process.

Responding means you think through what you want to have happen in an interaction or conflict. You are measured, thoughtful, and allow creative ideas to enter the process.

Reacting, on the other hand, is typically immediate, without thought, and often results in a negative outcome.

You question your thoughts.

The latest scientific research finds that the average person has more than six thousand thoughts every day. The next time a thought challenges your emotional well-being, follow a pattern by self-inquiry and ask yourself these four questions:

Is it true? Consider whether the thought reflects how you really feel. For example, if you think, "My life is a disaster right now," consider whether you truly feel that way.

Is it absolutely true? Go deeper, open your mind, and question what you think you know. If, after the first question, you thought, "Yes, my life is truly a disaster," consider why you think that. Are there perhaps just a few things you could change, and can you find some things are going well?

How do I feel when I think that thought? Consider the emotions and feelings that come along with a negative thought. For example, when you think your life is a disaster, you might feel hopeless, anxious, or melancholy.

Who would I be without that thought? Now, imagine your life without that negative thought. For example, you might be happier, more motivated, and more focused if you thought your life was wonderful. Consider which thoughts and feelings you prefer and make a conscious decision to focus on that.

To wrap up this practice, use the final step of turning around the initial thought that challenged your well-being. Come up with three reasons why your new thought might be true. The practice of questioning and then turning your thoughts around offers you a concrete way to return to a state of emotional well-being.

How can you improve your emotional well-being? Your range of emotions—and how you manage them— influences your emotional health. Here are eight ways you can control your emotions and feelings, and stay resilient:

1. Move your body. Do some sort of physical activity every 90 minutes. Exercise, yoga, stretching. Clean up your room. Weather permitting, get outside. Gardening or watering plants. Walk around the block. Run. Visit a park.

2. Establish a routine. Create a schedule that balances the work you do with the life you want. Set time for your meetings. Block space to set goals. Create room to read. Listen to music.

3. Connect with others. Love your family. Check in with those who support you. Ask for help. Learn something out of your comfort zone. Spend time with someone whom you respect.

4. Forgive. Forgive others and forgive yourself. Forgiveness frees you to keep your power. Forgiveness opens the path to live in the moment. Forgiveness allows for growth and happiness. It saves you from the toxin load of cortisol and calms down your mind.

5. Do something for others. Offer to do something for someone you know or don't know. Spend time with your grandchildren. Volunteer online. Send a thank-you note.

6. Sleep. Healthy sleep gives your body the chance to repair itself. Sleep refreshes your brain to manage your memories and process information. You wake up in a better mood.

7. Be kind to yourself. What gives you joy? Where are you most at peace? When do you have space to be you? As you are kind to yourself, you will want to extend that kindness beyond yourself.

8. Be self-aware. Notice the thoughts, actions, habits, and character traits that serve you well. And when you spot what needs to change, you'll be ready. You will simply know.

Final thoughts on emotional well-being: "Watch your thoughts; they become words. Watch your words; they become actions. Watch your actions; they become habits. Watch your habits; they become character. Watch your character; it becomes your destiny." - Lao Tzu

You become more resilient as you encounter and master any situation. Whenever you have doubts, and you will, remember that you have everything you need to take care of your emotional well-being. You will bounce back.

ManAgeing stress, anxiety, and depression in later life: ManAgeing stress, anxiety, and depression in later life is crucial for maintaining mental and emotional well-being and ensuring a fulfilling and vibrant Ageing journey. As seniors navigate the challenges and transitions of Ageing, they may encounter stressors related to health concerns, changes in lifestyle, loss of loved ones, or social isolation. Additionally, age-related factors such as declining physical health or cognitive changes can contribute to feelings of anxiety or depression. In this section, we explore effective strategies for manAgeing stress, anxiety, and depression in later life:

1. Recognize and Acknowledge Feelings: The first step in manAgeing stress, anxiety, or depression is to recognize and acknowledge the feelings that arise. One very powerful technique is to name the feeling and live through it by talking to yourself if anything can be done about it. If yes then definitely work on it. If it's something not in control then don't worry. I learned a pearl of wisdom from my father-in-law. He used to say- "Every difficult life situation can be an excuse for hopelessness or an opportunity for growth, depending on what you choose to do with it right now," my father-in-law told me. "We have to let go of the ideas, outcomes, and expectations that aren't serving us." They should allow themselves to experience their emotions without judgment and understand that it's normal to feel stressed or anxious at times, especially during significant life changes or challenges.

2. Write a Journal: Writing a journal is also a powerful technique to release and reduce stored past concerns and negative emotions. It helps you delve into that emotion and understand its deep purpose. For example, being sad is an emotion that may arise from feeling lonely. So when you engage with the emotion, talk to yourself, and ask what should be done to alleviate it. You will get an answer from your inner self. This is my experience with a number of people.

3. Practice Relaxation Techniques: Seniors can incorporate relaxation techniques into their daily routine to alleviate stress and promote a sense of calmness. Deep breathing exercises, progressive muscle relaxation, guided imagery, or meditation can help them reduce tension and anxiety levels, enhance relaxation, and improve overall well-being.

4. Engage in Physical Activity: Regular physical activity is an effective way to manage stress, anxiety, and depression in later life. Seniors can engage in activities such as walking, swimming, yoga, or tai chi to release endorphins, improve mood, and reduce feelings of stress or tension. Even moderate exercise can have significant benefits for mental and emotional well-being. We have already read in detail about the positive connection between exercise and emotions.

5. Nurturing Social Connections: Social support is essential for manAgeing stress and promoting mental health in later life. Seniors should prioritize maintaining relationships with friends, family members, or support groups who provide emotional support, companionship, and encouragement. Regular social interactions can help seniors feel connected, valued, and supported, reducing feelings of loneliness or isolation.

6. Seek Professional Help: If stress, anxiety, or depression become overwhelming or interfere with daily functioning, seniors should not hesitate to seek professional help. Mental health professionals, such as therapists or counselors, can provide guidance, support, and evidence-based interventions to help seniors manage their symptoms and improve their quality of life. Additionally, healthcare providers can offer medication or other treatments if necessary.

7. Practice Self-Care: Seniors should prioritize self-care practices that nurture their mental and emotional well-being. This may include activities such as spending time in nature, pursuing hobbies or interests, practicing gratitude, forgiveness, or mindfulness, or engAgeing in creative outlets. Seniors should make time for activities that bring them joy, fulfillment, and a sense of purpose. Gratitude and forgiveness practices are very powerful techniques to have relief from pent-up negative emotions and feelings which were a big burden on your heart and were not letting you live happily or express yourself.

By implementing these strategies and seeking support when needed, seniors can effectively manage stress, anxiety, and depression in later life and cultivate a greater sense of resilience, positivity, and emotional well-being. Along with manAgeing negative mental thoughts and feelings, it's important to cultivate positive emotional strength.

Fostering Resilience, Positivity, and Emotional Balance

Fostering resilience, positivity, and emotional balance is essential for seniors to navigate the challenges and transitions of Ageing with grace, strength, and a sense of well-being. Resilience enables individuals to bounce back from adversity, while positivity and emotional balance promote a greater sense of happiness and contentment in life. In this section, we explore effective strategies for fostering resilience, positivity, and emotional balance in seniors:

1. Cultivate a Positive Mindset

Seniors can cultivate a positive mindset by focusing on the present moment and embracing an attitude of gratitude. Practicing daily affirmations, keeping a gratitude journal, or reflecting on past achievements and blessings can help seniors maintain a positive outlook on life, even in the face of challenges or setbacks.

2. Embrace Change and Adaptability

Ageing often brings changes and transitions that can be challenging to navigate. Seniors can foster resilience by embracing change and viewing it as an opportunity for growth and self-discovery. Adopting a flexible and adaptable mindset allows seniors to approach life's changes with courage, openness, and resilience.

3. Develop Coping Strategies

Seniors can develop effective coping strategies to manage stress and adversity in healthy ways. This may include practicing relaxation techniques such as deep breathing, meditation, or progressive muscle relaxation to reduce stress levels and promote emotional balance. Additionally, engAgeing in hobbies, creative activities, or physical exercise can provide a healthy outlet for manAgeing emotions and enhancing well-being.

4. Build a Support Network

Social support is a powerful resource for fostering resilience and emotional well-being in seniors. Seniors should cultivate meaningful relationships with friends, family members, or support groups who provide encouragement, empathy, and companionship. Regular social interactions can help seniors feel connected, valued, and supported, reducing feelings of loneliness or isolation.

5. Practice Self-Compassion

Seniors should practice self-compassion and kindness toward themselves, especially during times of difficulty or challenge. Instead of being self-critical or judgmental, seniors should treat themselves with the same kindness and understanding they would offer to a friend facing similar circumstances. Self-compassion fosters resilience, emotional balance, and a greater sense of self-worth and acceptance.

6. Engage in Meaningful Activities

Seniors can enhance emotional well-being by engAgeing in activities that bring joy, fulfillment, and a sense of purpose. This may include pursuing hobbies or interests, volunteering in the community, or participating in activities that promote social connection and engagement. Meaningful activities provide opportunities for self-expression, creativity, and personal growth, enhancing overall well-being and satisfaction with life.

By fostering resilience, positivity, and emotional balance, seniors can navigate the ups and downs of Ageing with greater ease and confidence, leading to a more fulfilling and vibrant life. Through a combination of positive mindset, coping strategies, social support, and meaningful activities, seniors can cultivate greater resilience, emotional well-being, and overall quality of life as they age.

Strategies for Cognitive Health and Memory Maintenance:

Though slow cognitive decline is a natural process of Ageing of brain cells and neurons, with optimal physical care, nourishment, and mental exercises, cognitive health can be maintained in a much better way. It is essential for seniors to live independently and enjoy a high quality of life. There are several evidence-based strategies seniors can incorporate into their daily routines to promote brain health and reduce the risk of cognitive decline.

1. Physical Activity:

As mentioned earlier in the book, regular exercise has been shown to benefit cognitive function by improving blood flow to the brain, promoting the growth of new brain cells (neurogenesis), and reducing the risk of conditions such as dementia. Seniors should aim for a combination of aerobic exercise, strength training, and flexibility exercises to reap the maximum cognitive benefits. I have already mentioned the benefits of physical activity for mental well-being.

2. Mental Stimulation:

EngAgeing in mentally stimulating activities such as reading, puzzles, learning new skills, or playing musical instruments helps keep the brain active and sharp. It's essential to challenge the brain with novel tasks to promote neuroplasticity and cognitive resilience. For example, going for a morning walk on unfamiliar paths will stimulate your brain to take every step mindfully.

3. Healthy Diet:

A balanced and nutritious diet rich in fruits, vegetables, whole grains, lean proteins, and healthy fats provides essential nutrients that support brain health. Certain foods, such as those high in antioxidants (e.g., berries, leafy greens) and omega-3 fatty acids (e.g., fatty fish, flaxseeds), have been associated with improved cognitive function and memory.

4. Quality Sleep:

Adequate sleep is crucial for cognitive function, memory consolidation, and overall brain health. Seniors should prioritize good sleep hygiene practices, such as maintaining a regular sleep schedule, creating a comfortable sleep environment, and avoiding stimulants like caffeine or electronics before bedtime.

5. Social Engagement:

Staying socially active and maintaining meaningful connections with friends, family, and community groups is essential for cognitive health. Social interaction stimulates the brain, enhances emotional well-being, and provides opportunities for intellectual engagement and learning.

6. Stress Management:

Chronic stress can negatively impact cognitive function and memory. Seniors should practice stress-reduction techniques such as mindfulness, meditation, deep breathing exercises, or progressive muscle relaxation to promote relaxation and mental clarity.

7. Puzzle Games:

Encourage older adults to tackle crossword puzzles, Sudoku, word searches, jigsaw puzzles, or brain teaser games. These activities challenge the mind, improve problem-solving skills, and enhance cognitive function.

8. Learning New Skills:

Encourage lifelong learning by exploring new hobbies or interests. Whether it's learning a musical instrument, taking up painting or drawing, trying out photography, or learning a new language, engAgeing in new activities stimulates the brain and promotes neuroplasticity.

9. Reading and Book Clubs:

Reading is an excellent way to stimulate the mind and expand knowledge. Encourage older adults to read books, newspapers, magazines, or online articles on topics of interest. Participating in a book club provides opportunities for social interaction, discussion, and shared learning experiences.

10. Memory Games and Brain Training Apps:

There are numerous brain training apps and games specifically designed to improve memory, attention, and cognitive skills. Encourage older adults to use these apps regularly to challenge their minds and track their progress.

11. Music and Dance:

Listening to music, playing musical instruments, or dancing are enjoyable activities that stimulate the brain and promote emotional well-being. Encourage older adults to create playlists of their favorite songs, attend concerts or music events, or participate in dance classes or social dances.

12. Mindfulness and Meditation:

Practicing mindfulness and meditation techniques can help older adults reduce stress, improve focus, and enhance cognitive function. Encourage them to try guided meditation apps, mindfulness exercises, or relaxation techniques to promote mental well-being.

13. Socializing and Games:

EngAgeing in social activities and games with friends and family is a fun way to stimulate the mind and maintain social connections. Encourage older adults to play board games, card games, or group trivia games that require problem-solving, memory, and strategic thinking.

14. Gardening and Nature Activities:

Spending time outdoors in nature has been shown to improve cognitive function and reduce stress. Encourage older adults to engage in gardening, birdwatching, nature walks, or outdoor activities that promote sensory stimulation and connection with the natural world.

15. Volunteering and Community Engagement:

Volunteering in the community or participating in meaningful activities that give back to others promotes a sense of purpose, fulfillment, and social connection. Encourage older adults to volunteer at local organizations, mentor younger generations, or participate in community events and initiatives.

By incorporating these mental stimulation activities into their daily lives, older adults can promote vibrant Ageing, maintain cognitive function, and enjoy a higher quality of life as they age. Encourage them to stay curious, explore new interests, and engage in activities that challenge and inspire them intellectually.

MIND MAP

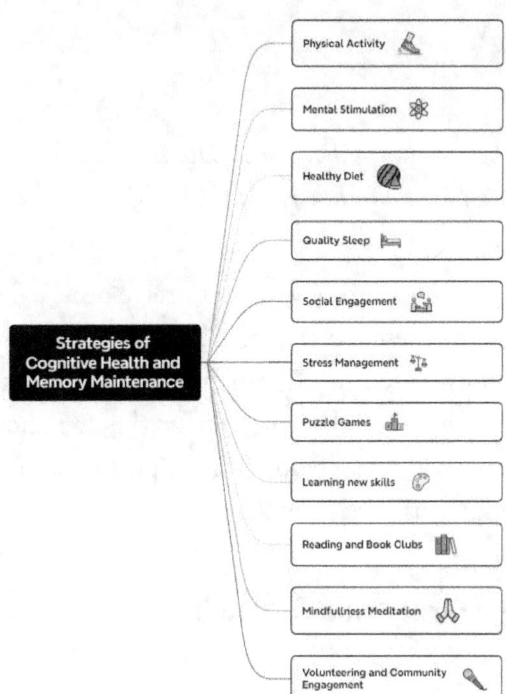

POWER OF GRATITUDE

Expressing gratitude for everything you have in life is a very powerful technique to elevate emotional and mental wellbeing.

"Gratitude is not only the greatest of virtues but the parent of all others." – Marcus Tullius Cicero

Discover more joy in your life through gratitude in everyday situations. Gratitude journaling is all about adding kinesthetic energy to the joy of expressing thanks for the abundance already in your life and for whatever is coming your way.

"Acknowledging the good that you already have in your life is the foundation for abundance." - Eckhart Tolle

Express gratitude for every opportunity you get to serve others. This will boost your well-being. These days, lives are getting busier and more stressful the older we become. It can be hard to start the day out in a positive mood and feel energized for the day ahead. Writing a gratitude journal will infuse you with the positive vitamin of abundance and be happy with what you have.

Benefits of writing a Gratitude Journal:

- Improves sleep

- Enhances mental well-being

- Increases empathy and compassion

- Reduces stress

- Builds social connections

- Enhances self-esteem

GUIDELINES TO WRITE A GRATITUDE JOURNAL:

You don't need a special skill or have an extraordinary experience to write in your journal. Simply acknowledge goodness in everyday situations. Appreciate all good things, no matter how small or simple—nothing is too small to be thankful for. Be thankful for difficult situations and failures and how they helped you become a better person you are today. Visualize things you are grateful for and experience the feelings of gratitude within your body.

Share and express your gratitude by writing in your gratitude journal every morning for whatever you have which is making your life better. It can also be written for whatever your future desires are. Visualize that happening now and write it down in your gratitude journal with full emotion.

"I AM SO HAPPY AND GRATEFUL FOR..."

- I am blessed with a wonderful family supporting me in all times of need.

- Opportunities for serving as a guide to my community.

- Learnings: the powerful strategies and practices to elevate my health.

- Friends and family

- Teachers and gurus

- Services

- Environment

- Health

- Nutrition

- Memories

- What I look forward to

- What I learned

- Emotions I felt

- DAILY REVIEW: Before sleeping, write in your journal 3 good things that happened that day and express your gratitude to God.

Also, write down about negative emotions and reactions. For example, if you have been complaining about every small thing around you. This becomes a route for venting out what was suppressed inside you. And how it leads to the release of harmful chemicals inside you. Moreover, it spoils your relationships and leads to stress. Once you review your journal, you get insight into the impact of your reactive behavior on your behavior and attitude. This helps you to adopt rectifying strategies to stay in a more balanced behavior. With a positive mindset, you become more resilient.

6

Nurturing Social Connections for Vibrant Aging

*"Good friends, good books, and a sleepy conscience: this is
the ideal life." - Mark Twain*

This quote by Mark Twain highlights the importance of social connections and relationships in leading a fulfilling and vibrant life. It emphasizes the value of meaningful friendships and human connection, suggesting that they contribute significantly to overall well-being and happiness, especially in later life.

"Social connections are the elixir of life, enriching our days and adding vibrancy to our years." They foster a sense of belonging and combat loneliness and isolation.

As individuals age, maintaining meaningful relationships and staying socially engaged become increasingly important for mental, emotional, and physical health. It's instrumental in reducing the risk of depression and anxiety and enhancing overall quality of life in seniors. Social connection, as I visualize it, is like a playground where we all play and have fun. We feel happy and refueled with more energy and enthusiasm for the rest of the day.

Just visualize your childhood when we used to play holding each other's hands - "Ring around the roses, pocket full of posies." This simple game used to fill us with immense pleasure in falling down together and then getting up for the repeat. Similarly, today, when we play, learn, share, and express to family, friends, or the community, it works like therapy, releasing a surge of the happy hormone dopamine.

Let us all make an endeavor to be the reason for each other's shot of dopamine. I am sure this thought itself will release all stress and anxiety from your mind. Reach out to your neighbor to fill their bucket with happy hormones. In return, you will get a double surge of it in your body. Just get up and see the smile on your face after reading this.

A robust body of scientific evidence has shown that lacking social connection is an indicator of premature mortality comparable to many leading health indicators.

Effective Strategies for Nurturing Social Connections:

Stay Connected with Loved Ones: Seniors should prioritize staying connected with family members, friends, and loved ones through regular communication, visits, or virtual interactions. Sharing experiences, memories, and conversations with loved ones strengthens bonds and promotes emotional well-being. Celebrating birthdays, planning vacations, and celebrating family day are wonderful ways of connecting and spending quality time with family. Family values are a legacy inherited by younger members of the family.

Also, family members get in-person updates on each other's well-being and are better prepared to take proactive action whenever required.

Join Social Groups and Clubs: Seniors can expand their social network and meet new people by joining social groups, clubs, or community organizations based on their interests and hobbies. Whether it's a spiritual meeting, book club, gardening group, or volunteer organization, participating in group activities provides opportunities for social interaction, shared interests, mutual learning, and meaningful connections.

Volunteer in the Community: Volunteering is a rewarding way for seniors to give back to the community while also fostering social connections and a sense of purpose. Seniors can volunteer at local charities, schools, hospitals, or community centers, contributing their time and skills to meaningful causes and building relationships with others who share similar values and interests. Participating actively in Resident Welfare associations gives seniors an opportunity to share their wisdom for WIN/WIN benefits for all the residents.

Attend Social Events and Activities: Seniors should take advantage of social events, festival celebrations, gatherings, and activities in their community to meet new people and engage in enjoyable experiences. Whether it's attending a lecture, concert, or fitness class, participating in social activities provides opportunities for interaction, laughter, and shared experiences with others.

Utilize Technology for Social Connection: Technology can be a valuable tool for staying connected with others, especially for seniors who may face mobility or transportation challenges. Seniors can use social media, video calls, or online forums to connect with friends, family members, and peers, reducing feelings of isolation and loneliness.

Seek Support when Needed: If seniors are experiencing feelings of loneliness or isolation, it's important to reach out for support from trusted friends, family members, or mental health professionals. Support groups, counseling services, or senior centers can provide valuable resources and opportunities for connection and support.

Benefits of Social Engagement and Meaningful Relationships for Seniors

The benefits of social engagement and meaningful relationships for seniors are profound and far-reaching.

Emotional Support: Meaningful relationships provide seniors with emotional support during times of stress, loss, or difficulty. Having trusted friends, family members, or peers to confide in and lean on can alleviate feelings of loneliness and isolation and promote emotional well-being.

Sense of Belonging: Social engagement fosters a sense of belonging and connectedness in seniors, reducing feelings of loneliness and enhancing overall quality of life. Being part of a social network or community gives seniors a sense of identity, purpose, and camaraderie.

Cognitive Stimulation: Social interactions stimulate the brain and promote cognitive function in seniors. EngAgeing in conversations, sharing stories, and participating in group activities challenge the mind and help seniors stay mentally sharp and agile.

Physical Health: Socially engaged seniors tend to have better physical health outcomes compared to those who are socially isolated. Research has shown that social connections are associated with lower rates of chronic diseases, better immune function, and improved longevity.

Reduced Risk of Depression and Anxiety: Meaningful relationships and social engagement act as protective factors against depression and anxiety in seniors. Regular social interactions provide opportunities for laughter, joy, and emotional support, helping seniors maintain a positive outlook on life.

Increased Resilience: Seniors who are socially engaged tend to be more resilient and better equipped to cope with life's challenges and stressors. Having a strong support network and meaningful relationships can buffer against the negative effects of adversity and promote emotional well-being.

Enhanced Quality of Life: Overall, social engagement and meaningful relationships contribute to a higher quality of life for seniors. By fostering connections with others, seniors experience greater happiness, fulfillment, and satisfaction with life, leading to a more vibrant and enjoyable Ageing journey.

By prioritizing social connections and nurturing meaningful relationships, seniors can experience emotional support, a sense of belonging, cognitive stimulation, improved physical health, reduced risk of depression and anxiety, increased resilience, and enhanced overall quality of life.

Through a commitment to staying socially engaged and fostering meaningful relationships, seniors can enjoy a fulfilling and vibrant

Ageing journey, surrounded by the love, support, and camaraderie of their social networks.

7

—— • ——

MANAGING CHRONIC CONDITIONS FOR VIBRANT AGING IN SENIORS

"Vibrant Ageing is not the absence of challenges, but the presence of resilience, adaptability, and a relentless spirit that refuses to be defined by chronic conditions."

With progressive years of life, there is a natural cycle of slowdown of the body's regeneration power. Throughout life, there is a continuous process of depletion of old cells and regeneration of new cells. But there is a very fine tuning between both processes. However, as we grow older, regeneration of new cells becomes slower compared to depletion of old cells. This also impacts the repairing process as well. Besides this, the metabolic process of our body slows down gradually with Ageing.

If you sell out to the natural cycle of declination and fall prey to complacent self-care, erratic lifestyle, inadequate nourishment, inactivity, anxiety, and worry, then the likelihood of developing chronic health conditions increases, presenting unique challenges that require proactive management and care.

Vibrant Ageing is adapting to changes of the natural cycle and being proactive in taking remedial measures to best live through these challenges on the route. Smart and mindful management of a purposeful life elevates wellness, boosts metabolism, and strengthens immunity. In this chapter, we delve into effective strategies for seniors to manage chronic conditions, maintain quality of life, and promote vibrant Ageing despite health challenges. The strategies suggested in earlier chapters for physical, emotional, and mental wellness will be very effective in smooth management of chronic conditions if any.

Coping with the challenges of manAgeing symptoms, adhering to treatment plans, and adjusting to lifestyle changes requires resilience and support. Seniors can benefit from developing coping strategies such as acceptance, self-care, and seeking social support from peers, caregivers, or support groups. Additionally, staying informed about their condition, communicating openly with healthcare providers, and actively participating in their treatment plan empowers seniors to take control of their health and well-being.

Strategies for Disease Management and Prevention:

Prevention and proactive management are the key components of effectively manAgeing chronic conditions in seniors. Seniors should prioritize preventive measures such as regular screenings, vaccinations, and lifestyle modifications to reduce the risk of disease progression and complications.

Refer to chapters 4-5 for implementing healthy habits for elevating wellness and manAgeing chronic conditions.

Despite living with chronic conditions, seniors can take steps to enhance their quality of life and maintain independence and vitality. This may involve incorporating adaptive strategies and assistive devices to overcome physical limitations and maintain functional independence. Seniors can also benefit from palliative care and symptom management strategies to alleviate pain, discomfort, and improve overall well-being. Additionally, fostering social connections, engAgeing in meaningful activities, and cultivating a positive outlook can enhance resilience and promote overall quality of life despite chronic health challenges. First of all, let's understand and be informed about the common chronic illnesses and age-related health conditions. The sole purpose of understanding is to gain knowledge and strategies of coping up well with any such challenge if a person happens to counter.

Understanding Common Chronic Illnesses and Age-Related Health Conditions:

As individuals age, they become more susceptible to various chronic illnesses and age-related health conditions that can significantly impact their quality of life. In this section, we explore some of the most common chronic illnesses and age-related health conditions that affect seniors, along with their symptoms, risk factors, and management strategies.

Cardiovascular Disease:

Cardiovascular disease encompasses a range of conditions that affect the heart and blood vessels, including coronary artery disease, hypertension (high blood pressure), and heart failure. Symptoms may include chest pain, shortness of breath, fatigue, and swelling in the legs. Risk factors for cardiovascular disease include age, family history, smoking, poor diet, lack of exercise, and obesity. Management strategies may include lifestyle modifications such as following a heart-healthy diet, exercising regularly, quitting smoking, manAgeing stress, and taking medications to control blood pressure and cholesterol levels.

Diabetes:

Diabetes is a chronic condition characterized by high blood sugar levels resulting from the body's inability to produce or effectively use insulin. Type 2 diabetes is more common in older adults and is often associated with obesity and sedentary lifestyles. Symptoms may include increased thirst, frequent urination, fatigue, and slow wound healing. Management strategies for diabetes include blood sugar monitoring, following a balanced diet, engAgeing in regular physical activity, taking medications as prescribed, and manAgeing stress levels.

Arthritis:

Arthritis is a group of conditions that cause inflammation and stiffness in the joints, leading to pain and decreased mobility. Osteoarthritis, rheumatoid arthritis, and gout are among the most common types of arthritis in seniors. Symptoms may include joint pain, stiffness, swelling, and difficulty with movement. Risk factors for arthritis include age, genetics, obesity, and joint injuries. Management strategies may include pain management techniques such as medications, physical therapy, exercise, weight management, and assistive devices to support joint function.

Osteoporosis:

Osteoporosis is a condition characterized by weakened bones that are more susceptible to fractures. It is more common in women than men, especially after menopause, due to hormonal changes that lead to bone loss. Symptoms may not be apparent until a fracture occurs, making early detection and prevention crucial. Risk factors for osteoporosis include age, gender, family history, low body weight, smoking, and lack of exercise. Management strategies may include calcium and vitamin D supplementation, weight-bearing exercise, fall prevention measures, and medications to slow bone loss.

Alzheimer's Disease and Dementia:

Alzheimer's disease and other forms of dementia are progressive neurological disorders that affect memory, cognitive function, and behavior. Symptoms may include memory loss, confusion, difficulty with language, and changes in mood or personality. Risk factors for Alzheimer's disease and dementia include age, family history, genetics, and certain lifestyle factors such as smoking and lack of physical activity. While there is no cure for Alzheimer's disease, management strategies may include medication to manage symptoms, cognitive stimulation activities, support from caregivers, and lifestyle modifications to promote brain health.

Conclusion:

Understanding common chronic illnesses and age-related health conditions is essential for seniors to effectively manage their health and well-being as they age. By recognizing the symptoms, risk factors, and management strategies for these conditions, seniors can take proactive steps to prevent or manage chronic illness, optimize their health, and maintain a high quality of life in their later years. Regular health screenings, adherence to treatment plans, and lifestyle modifications are key components of promoting healthy Ageing and longevity.

Adopting a healthy lifestyle is the key instrument in enjoying exuberant health throughout and Ageing vibrantly. Embracing vitality in old age is a testament to your lifelong commitment to wellness. By prioritizing health and well-being throughout adulthood, you lay the foundation for a vibrant and fulfilling later life. Your dedication to healthy habits, such as regular exercise, nutritious eating, and mindfulness, contributes to your physical resilience, mental sharpness, and emotional well-being as you age.

Embracing vitality in old age is not just a reward for your past efforts but a reflection of your sincere dedication to nurturing your body, mind, and spirit throughout your journey.

Tips for ManAgeing Symptoms, Reducing Complications, and Enhancing Quality of Life:

ManAgeing chronic conditions and age-related health concerns requires a proactive approach to care, focusing on symptom management, prevention of complications, and optimizing overall quality of life. Enlisted practical tips and strategies work like a compass to choose the right direction to effectively manage their symptoms, reduce the risk of complications, and enhance their quality of life.

Follow a Healthy Lifestyle:

Maintaining a healthy lifestyle is essential for manAgeing chronic conditions and promoting overall well-being. Seniors should focus on following a balanced diet rich in fruits, vegetables, whole grains, lean proteins, and healthy fats. Regular physical activity, such as walking, swimming, or tai chi, can help manage symptoms, improve mobility, and reduce the risk of complications. Additionally, avoiding tobacco, limiting alcohol consumption, and manAgeing stress through relaxation techniques or mindfulness practices can support overall health and well-being.

Adhere to Treatment Plans:

Consistently following prescribed treatment plans is critical for manAgeing chronic conditions and preventing complications. Seniors should take medications as prescribed by their healthcare provider, following dosing instructions and scheduling regular medication reviews. It's essential to communicate any concerns or side effects with healthcare providers to ensure treatment plans are effective and well-tolerated. In addition to medications, seniors should adhere to recommended lifestyle modifications, such as dietary changes, exercise routines, or monitoring blood sugar levels, to effectively manage their condition.

Monitor Symptoms and Progress:

Regular monitoring of symptoms and health status allows seniors to track changes in their condition and identify any potential complications early on. Seniors should be proactive in monitoring vital signs, blood sugar levels, or other relevant markers as advised by their healthcare provider. Keeping track of symptoms, changes in medication, or lifestyle modifications in a journal or health app can provide valuable information for healthcare providers and empower seniors to take an active role in manAgeing their health.

Communicate with Healthcare Providers:

Open and honest communication with healthcare providers is essential for effective symptom management and prevention of complications. Seniors should feel comfortable discussing any concerns, questions, or changes in their health with their healthcare team. Regular check-ups, screenings, and follow-up appointments provide opportunities for healthcare providers to assess health status, adjust treatment plans as needed, and address any emerging issues promptly.

Engage in Self-Care Practices:

Practicing self-care techniques can help seniors manage symptoms, reduce stress, and enhance overall well-being. Seniors can incorporate relaxation techniques such as deep breathing, meditation, or gentle stretching into their daily routine to promote relaxation and stress relief. EngAgeing in enjoyable activities, hobbies, or social interactions can provide a sense of joy, fulfillment, and connection, contributing to improved quality of life.

Seek Support from Loved Ones:

Support from family members, friends, and caregivers is invaluable for seniors manAgeing chronic conditions and age-related health concerns. Seniors should not hesitate to reach out for assistance or emotional support when needed. Having a strong support network provides encouragement, companionship, and practical assistance with daily tasks, reducing feelings of loneliness and enhancing overall well-being. It strengthens the relationship bond as well. Compassion and love automatically flow into life, which in itself is therapeutic and, in fact, heals at a faster rate.

By following these tips for manAgeing symptoms, reducing complications, and enhancing quality of life, seniors can take proactive steps to optimize their health and well-being as they age. By prioritizing healthy lifestyle habits, adhering to treatment plans, monitoring symptoms, communicating with healthcare providers, practicing self-care, and seeking support from loved ones, seniors can effectively manage chronic conditions and enjoy a fulfilling and vibrant life in their later years.

Empowering seniors to take charge of their health and advocate for their wellness needs is essential for promoting independence, autonomy, and overall well-being. In this section, we explore practical strategies and resources to empower seniors to actively engage in their healthcare and advocate for their wellness needs effectively.

Educate Yourself:

Knowledge is power, and seniors can empower themselves by educating themselves about their health conditions, treatment options, and available resources. Seniors should take the initiative to research their conditions, ask questions during medical appointments, and seek reliable information from trusted sources such as healthcare providers, reputable websites, or patient advocacy organizations. By understanding their health status and treatment options, seniors can make informed decisions about their care and advocate for their needs more effectively.

Communicate Effectively:

Effective communication with healthcare providers is crucial for seniors to advocate for their wellness needs. Seniors should feel comfortable expressing their concerns, asking questions, and seeking clarification about their health conditions, treatment plans, and medication regimens. It's essential to communicate openly and honestly with healthcare providers, providing detailed information about symptoms, concerns, or changes in health status to ensure accurate diagnosis and appropriate treatment.

Be Proactive in Healthcare:

Seniors should take a proactive approach to their healthcare by scheduling regular check-ups, screenings, and preventive services recommended by healthcare providers. By prioritizing preventive care and early intervention, seniors can identify health issues early on and take proactive steps to address them before they escalate. Seniors should also keep track of their medical history, medications, and test results, maintaining a personal health record to facilitate communication with healthcare providers and ensure continuity of care.

Advocate for Accessible Healthcare:

Seniors have the right to access high-quality, affordable healthcare services that meet their unique needs and preferences. For example, hospitals often have special Geriatric units to address old-age issues, and there are senior citizen facilities at various healthcare centers. Seniors should advocate for accessible healthcare by speaking up about barriers to care, such as transportation challenges, affordability issues, or limited access to specialized services. They can work with healthcare providers, community organizations, and policymakers to advocate for policies and initiatives that improve access to healthcare services and support systems for seniors.

Seek Support from Loved Ones:

Family members, friends, and caregivers can play a crucial role in empowering seniors to advocate for their wellness needs. Seniors should seek support from loved ones in navigating the healthcare system, attending medical appointments, and making informed decisions about their care. Having a trusted advocate or support system provides encouragement, emotional support, and practical assistance in manAgeing health challenges and advocating for wellness needs effectively.

Utilize Community Resources:

Seniors can access a variety of community resources and support services to help them advocate for their wellness needs. Community organizations, senior centers, and patient advocacy groups offer educational programs, support groups, and workshops on health-related topics, empowering seniors with knowledge, skills, and resources to navigate the healthcare system and advocate for their well-being effectively.

By empowering seniors to take charge of their health and advocate for their wellness needs, we can promote autonomy, independence, and dignity in Ageing. By educating themselves, communicating effectively, being proactive in healthcare, advocating for accessible healthcare, seeking support from loved ones, and utilizing community resources, seniors can assert their rights, make informed decisions about their care, and lead healthier, more fulfilling lives in their later years. Empowering seniors to advocate for their wellness needs not only enhances their quality of life but also promotes positive healthcare outcomes and ensures that their voices are heard and respected in the healthcare system.

8

Navigating Healthcare and Wellness Resources for Seniors

Navigating the complex landscape of healthcare and wellness resources can be daunting for seniors. In this chapter, we explore strategies and tips for seniors to access healthcare services, insurance options, and support networks effectively. Additionally, we provide guidance on communicating with healthcare providers and navigating the healthcare system with confidence.

Accessing Healthcare Services, Insurance Options, and Support Networks for Seniors:

Understand Healthcare Options: Seniors should familiarize themselves with available healthcare options, including private insurance plans and government assistance programs. Understanding eligibility criteria, coverage options, and enrollment processes can help seniors make informed decisions about their healthcare coverage.

Enroll in Health Insurance Company: For seniors aged 65 and older, enrolling in a suitable Health Insurance company is essential for accessing healthcare services. Be in touch with your nearest healthcare agent and understand the various policies suitable for you.

Seek Help from Organizations and Initiatives: Several organizations and initiatives are dedicated to providing elderly care services in India. Here are some examples:

- **HelpAge India:** A non-profit organization dedicated to serving the needs of senior citizens across India. Established in 1978, HelpAge India works towards improving the quality of life and advocating for the rights of older adults.

- **Dignity Foundation:** Focuses on enhancing the quality of life for senior citizens in India by offering health camps, recreational activities, skill development programs, and advocacy initiatives.

- **Nightingales Medical Trust:** Provides healthcare and support services for senior citizens, including home healthcare services, geriatric clinics, and rehabilitation programs.

- **Silver Innings:** Specializes in providing support and advocacy for senior citizens and their families, addressing issues related to Ageing, dementia, and elder abuse.

HelpAge India's Mobile Healthcare Units: Operates mobile healthcare units in various parts of the country to provide medical care and support services to older adults in remote and underserved areas.

Elders Helpline: Several cities in India have established elders helplines to provide assistance, support, and referrals for senior citizens in need.

Tips for Communicating with Healthcare Providers and Navigating the Healthcare System:

Prepare for Medical Appointments: Seniors should prepare for medical appointments by writing down questions, concerns, and symptoms beforehand. Bringing a list of medications, medical history, and insurance information can facilitate communication with healthcare providers.

Advocate for Your Needs: Seniors should advocate for their healthcare needs by communicating openly and assertively with healthcare providers. Asking questions, seeking clarification, and expressing concerns can help seniors make informed decisions about their care.

Utilize Health Information Resources: Seniors can access reliable health information resources, such as reputable websites and patient education materials, to learn more about their conditions, treatment options, and available support services.

Keep Records and Follow-Up: Seniors should keep records of medical appointments, test results, medications, and treatment plans to track their healthcare journey effectively. Following up with healthcare providers and staying proactive in manAgeing their health can help seniors achieve optimal health outcomes.

Navigating healthcare and wellness resources can empower seniors to access essential services, advocate for their healthcare needs, and navigate the healthcare system with confidence. By understanding healthcare options, enrolling in appropriate coverage, seeking support networks, preparing for medical appointments, advocating for their needs, utilizing health information resources, and keeping records, seniors can take control of their health and well-being in their later years. Effective communication with healthcare providers and proactive engagement in healthcare decision-making are essential for promoting positive health outcomes and ensuring that seniors receive the care and support they deserve.

9

CREATING A PERSONAL WELLNESS PLAN

"Embrace vibrant Ageing; let plans propel dreams into radiant reality."

*E*mbark on your journey visualizing the possibility, empowering your potential, transforming your life.

Creating a personal wellness plan is a proactive approach to optimizing your health, happiness, and overall well-being. Here's a step-by-step guide to help you create your own personalized wellness plan:

Assess Your Current Lifestyle:

Create a personal journal and write down your assessment.

Take stock of your current habits and lifestyle choices related to physical activity, nutrition, sleep, stress management, social connections, and self-care.

Identify areas where you're doing well and areas where you'd like to make improvements and what you will do to make improvement.

Set Specific Goals: Based on your assessment, set specific, measurable, achievable, relevant, and time-bound (SMART) goals for each aspect of wellness you want to address. For example, you might set a goal to exercise or do yoga for 30 minutes five days a week, eat at least five servings of fruits and vegetables daily, write down your gratitude journal, or practice meditation for 10 minutes each day.

Identify Strategies and Actions: Brainstorm strategies and actions you can take to achieve your wellness goals. This might include joining a yoga or fitness class, meal planning and preparation, establishing a bedtime routine for better sleep, practicing relaxation techniques such as deep breathing or yoga, scheduling regular social outings, and prioritizing self-care activities such as reading, hobbies, or creative pursuits.

Prioritize Self-Care: Recognize the importance of self-care in your wellness plan. Make time for activities that nourish your body, mind, and spirit, such as exercise, relaxation, hobbies, spending time with loved ones, and pursuing personal interests. Prioritizing self-care helps you recharge, reduce stress, and maintain a sense of balance and well-being.

Create a Routine: Develop a daily or weekly routine that incorporates your wellness goals and activities. Schedule specific times for waking up, personal affirmations, exercise, breathing exercises, reading books, writing gratitude journal, relaxation or meditation, socializing, volunteering for social causes, meal planning, calm meal times, reflecting on your day before sleeping, and self-care to ensure consistency and accountability. Establishing a routine helps you stay on track and make your wellness habits a regular part of your life.

Track Your Progress: Keep track of your progress towards your wellness goals by monitoring your actions, behaviors, and outcomes. Use tools such as a journal, planner, or mobile app to record your daily activities, achievements, challenges, and reflections. It can be done on paper with a pen or digitally. But penning it down yourself adds in kinesthetic energy. Tracking your progress helps you stay motivated, identify areas for improvement, and celebrate your successes along the way.

Adjust and Adapt: Be flexible and open to adjusting your wellness plan as needed based on your evolving needs, preferences, and circumstances. If you encounter obstacles or setbacks, don't get discouraged—instead, reassess your goals, revise your strategies, and seek support from friends, family, or professionals if necessary. Remember that wellness is a journey, and it's okay to take detours or change course as you navigate your path.

Celebrate Your Success: Celebrate your progress and achievements as you work towards your wellness goals. Acknowledge the positive changes you've made, no matter how small, and reward yourself for your efforts. Celebrating your success reinforces your commitment to wellness and motivates you to continue striving for improvement. Rewarding is a beautiful motivator and kicks in dopamine. Happiness flows from your inner soul.

By following these steps and creating a personalized wellness plan, you can take charge of your health and well-being and embark on a journey towards a happier, healthier, and more fulfilling life.

MIND MAP

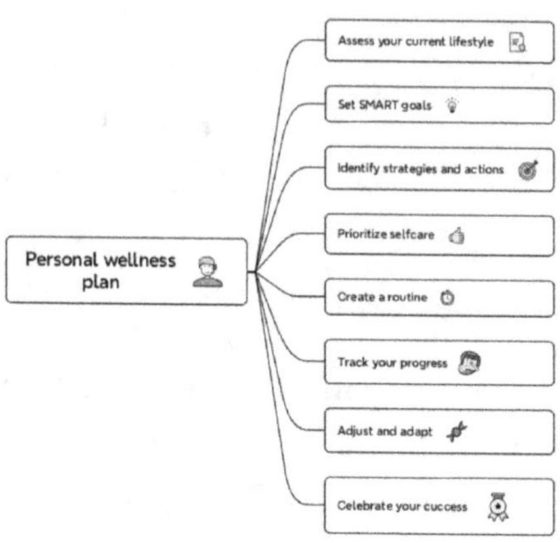

Visualization

Are you wondering how to actualize what you want in your life? How to transform your dreams into reality? Visualization is a powerful process to achieve your goals. After crafting a personalized plan, we need to create its manifestation in our minds. This is true for anything we want to achieve: we first imagine, plan, and visualize from action to end result in our minds. The second step is to actually take action when we are sure that this is what we have to do to achieve desirable results. Similarly, once you've determined the "why" and what you want for sustaining your physical, emotional, and wellness, and how you will attain your goal, you chalk out the action plan, and you are ready to implement and take action. The tool to empower your "how" is visualization.

Follow these simple steps to visualize every day to attain your micro goal:

1. Sit Comfortably: Sit comfortably and do silent deep breathing with awareness, which calms your mind and body.

2. Say Your Personalized Affirmation: Say your personalized affirmation which empowers your capability.

3. Imagine Your Goal Being Attained: Visualize yourself in the moment when you have accomplished your target and feel the emotion which rises within you. Visualization is simply imagining the moment and experiencing the feeling of fulfillment of your inner desires, your goal. It's the energy of this feeling which infuses you with motivation, courage, and confidence to tread the path towards your goal.

The 4 C Formula for success is empowered with VISUALIZATION:

- Commitment

- Courage

- Capability

- Confidence

So after being silent with deep breathing for a few minutes, say your affirmations in a power pose and then visualize your life unfolding in your inner eye. And there you experience miracles twinkling all around in your life.

Once you have chalked a crystal clear action plan to take you towards your goal of wellness, the goal of Ageing vibrantly, the goal of adding value to the society you live in, the goal of living life with a purpose, visualize it clearly happening in real.

As Ralph Waldo Emerson once said, "The purpose of life is not simply to be happy. It is to be useful, to be honorable, to be compassionate, to have it make some difference that you have lived and lived well."

"Anything you can imagine, you can create." - Oprah Winfrey

Conclusion: Unlocking Your Full Potential

As we conclude this guide to senior wellness, it's important to reflect on the journey we've taken together and the possibilities that lie ahead. Ageing is not merely a process of decline but an opportunity to unlock your full potential and embrace a life of purpose, vitality, and fulfillment. In this conclusion, we will explore key themes and insights from this guide, offer encouragement and inspiration for the road ahead, and provide practical tips for continuing your journey toward holistic wellness and personal growth.

REFLECTING ON THE JOURNEY OF VIBRANT AGING AND PERSONAL GROWTH

Reflecting on the journey of vibrant Ageing and personal growth is an opportunity to gain insights, appreciate progress, and set intentions for the future. Here's how to engage in meaningful reflection:

1. Acknowledge Your Progress: Take a moment to acknowledge how far you've come on your journey of vibrant Ageing and personal growth. Celebrate the milestones you've reached, the challenges you've overcome, and the lessons you've learned along the way. Recognize your resilience, determination, and commitment to living a vibrant and fulfilling life.

2. Identify Areas of Growth: Reflect on the areas of your life where you've experienced significant growth and transformation. Consider how you've evolved physically, mentally, emotionally, socially, and spiritually over time. Identify the skills you've developed, the beliefs you've challenged, and the values you've embraced on your journey towards vibrant Ageing and personal fulfillment.

3. Learn from Challenges and Setbacks: Reflect on the challenges and setbacks you've encountered on your path to vibrant Ageing. Consider how these experiences have shaped you, taught you valuable lessons, and strengthened your resilience. Identify the strategies and coping mechanisms you've used to navigate difficult times and overcome obstacles with grace and perseverance.

4. Celebrate Moments of Joy and Gratitude: Take time to reflect on the moments of joy, fulfillment, and gratitude you've experienced along the way. Recall the relationships, experiences, and achievements that have brought meaning and purpose to your life. Cultivate a sense of gratitude for the blessings you've received and the opportunities you've been given to thrive and grow.

5. Set Intentions for the Future: Use reflection as an opportunity to set intentions for the future and clarify your vision for vibrant Ageing and continued personal growth. Consider the goals, aspirations, and dreams you have for yourself in the years ahead. Set clear intentions for how you want to nurture your health, relationships, passions, and sense of purpose as you continue on your journey.

6. Commit to Ongoing Learning and Development: Embrace reflection as a catalyst for ongoing learning and development. Stay curious, open-minded, and receptive to new ideas, experiences, and perspectives. Seek out opportunities for personal and professional growth that align with your interests and values. Cultivate a mindset of lifelong learning and continuous improvement as you age gracefully.

7. Practice Self-Compassion and Acceptance: Be gentle with yourself as you reflect on your journey of vibrant Ageing and personal growth. Embrace your imperfections, vulnerabilities, and limitations with compassion and acceptance. Recognize that growth often involves

setbacks and challenges, and that self-compassion is essential for resilience and well-being.

8. Express Gratitude and Share Your Wisdom: Take time to express gratitude for the lessons learned, the growth experienced, and the blessings received on your journey. Share your wisdom, insights, and experiences with others, whether through writing, mentoring, or community involvement. By sharing your journey with others, you contribute to the collective wisdom and inspire others to embrace vibrant Ageing and personal growth.

In conclusion, reflection is a powerful tool for deepening self-awareness, appreciating progress, and setting intentions for the future on the journey of vibrant Ageing and personal growth. By engAgeing in regular reflection, you can cultivate resilience, gratitude, and a sense of purpose as you continue to evolve and thrive throughout life's journey.

My Message to the Readers From the Core of My Heart

I am one of you all, on the journey of vibrant Ageing. I am soon going to complete the sixth decade of my life. My mission is to encourage, inspire, and empower one million senior citizens to unleash their full potential and thrive in this beautiful journey of life, living happy, healthy, prosperous, and spiritually fulfilled lives.

Dear Reader,

As you continue on your journey through life, I want to remind you of the immense potential that lies within you to embrace wellness, vitality, and purpose in your later years. Despite the challenges and uncertainties that may come your way, know that you possess the strength, resilience, and wisdom to navigate life's twists and turns with grace and determination.

Embrace Wellness: Your health and well-being are precious gifts that deserve your utmost care and attention. Nurture your body, mind, and spirit through nourishing foods, regular exercise, restful sleep, and mindfulness practices. Prioritize self-care and make time for activities that bring you joy, relaxation, and rejuvenation. Remember that small, consistent steps towards wellness can yield significant benefits over time.

Cultivate Vitality: Age is not a barrier to vitality; it is an opportunity to embrace life with renewed energy and enthusiasm. Engage in activities that ignite your passions, stimulate your creativity, and challenge your mind. Stay curious, adventurous, and open to new experiences. Surround yourself with positive influences, supportive relationships, and a vibrant community that uplifts and inspires you. Embrace each day as a gift and seize every opportunity to live fully and authentically.

Discover Purpose: Your life has meaning and purpose, and your unique gifts and talents have the power to make a positive impact in the world. Reflect on what brings you fulfillment and align your actions with your values and aspirations. Find ways to contribute to causes that are meaningful to you, whether through volunteering, mentoring, or advocacy. Embrace opportunities for personal growth, learning, and self-discovery, and allow your journey to unfold with purpose and intention.

Remember, age is just a number, and there is no expiration date on your dreams, ambitions, or potential. Embrace each day as a new opportunity to thrive, grow, and make a difference in the world. Your journey of wellness, vitality, and purpose is a testament to your resilience, courage, and unwavering spirit. Embrace it wholeheartedly, and let your light shine brightly for all to see.

With love and encouragement,
Uma Gupta

May this message serve as a source of inspiration and motivation to continue embracing wellness, vitality, and purpose in the later years of life.

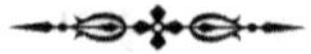

Final Thoughts, Resources, and Inspiration for Seniors to Unleash Their Full Potential

Dear Seniors,

As you embark on your journey of self-discovery and personal growth, I want to leave you with some final thoughts, resources, and inspiration to help you unleash your full potential and live your best life:

Believe in Yourself: Remember that age is not a limitation; it's an opportunity. Believe in your abilities, strengths, and resilience. Trust that you have the wisdom, experience, and inner strength to overcome any obstacle and achieve your dreams. Your belief auto suggests to subconscious mind to manifest what you desire. So believing in yourself forecasts your life's events.

Stay Curious and Open-Minded: Embrace a mindset of lifelong learning and exploration. Stay curious, open-minded, and receptive to new ideas, experiences, and perspectives. Keep seeking knowledge, trying new things, and stepping outside of your comfort zone.

Embrace Change and Growth: Embrace change as a natural part of life and view it as an opportunity for growth and transformation. Be willing to adapt, evolve, and reinvent yourself as you navigate the challenges and opportunities of Ageing. Embrace the journey of self-discovery and personal growth with courage and resilience.

Celebrate Your Accomplishments: Take time to celebrate your accomplishments, no matter how small. Recognize and honor the progress you've made, the challenges you've overcome, and the milestones you've reached along the way. Celebrate your resilience, perseverance, and unwavering spirit.

Seek Support and Connection: Surround yourself with a supportive community of friends, family members, and mentors who uplift and inspire you. Seek out resources, support groups, and organizations that cater to the needs and interests of seniors. Stay connected, engaged, and involved in activities that bring you joy and fulfillment.

Find Purpose and Meaning: Discover what brings you purpose, fulfillment, and meaning in life. Reflect on your passions, values, and aspirations, and align your actions with your deepest desires. Find ways to contribute to the well-being of others and make a positive impact in your community and the world.

Practice Gratitude and Mindfulness: Cultivate a daily practice of gratitude and mindfulness to foster a sense of peace, contentment, and joy in your life. Take time to appreciate the blessings, beauty, and abundance that surround you each day. Stay present, mindful, and fully engaged in the richness of each moment.

Stay Active and Engaged: Stay physically active, mentally engaged, and socially connected to maintain your vitality and well-being. Engage in regular exercise, hobbies, and activities that bring you joy and fulfillment. Stay connected with friends, family members, and your community to combat loneliness and isolation.

Remember, you have the power to create a life of purpose, passion, and fulfillment at any age. Seize the moment, embrace the journey, and unleash your full potential with courage, confidence, and determination.

With warmest wishes for a life filled with health, happiness, and boundless possibilities,

Uma Gupta

May these final thoughts, resources, and inspiration serve as a guiding light on your journey of self-discovery, personal growth, and vibrant living.

MIND MAP

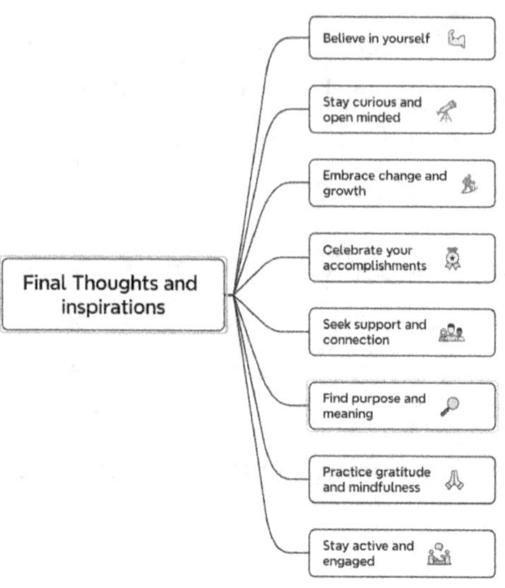

My father's journey:

I would like to share my father's journey briefly.

My father, Late Sh. Kewal Krishan, was diagnosed with diabetes at the age of 50. Initially, he was perturbed by the diagnosis, but his resilient nature and confidence in his abilities motivated him to tackle this challenge and reverse the numbers.

He created a wellness plan and began going for regular morning walks with enthusiasm to Baradari Garden in the heart of Patiala city. Not only did he enjoy his walks every morning, but he also looked forward to meeting a group of fellow morning walkers. They named their group "Haso aur hasao," which means "Laugh and make everyone laugh."

With the motive to radiate happiness and laughter, the group started growing in number. This served as therapy for many, providing emotional support.

After completing his 45-minute walk in the lush green gardens filled with fruit trees and vibrant floral beds, inhaling therapeutic floral fragrances, and with his heart elated by the sweet music of birds chirping, they all would gather on the central platform in the garden. There, they practiced yoga, laughed out loud, and shared sorrows and joys of their lives with each other. They also exchanged tips on natural therapies.

He used to return with Motiya flowers carefully collected in his pocket, radiating happiness. He would then carefully arrange these flowers in a vase on the dining table.

Not only did he live vibrantly until the ripe age of 91, manAgeing his diabetes and other implications of old age resiliently, but he also left a legacy behind in the form of words of wisdom with his children. I have shared those pearls of wisdom in this book in various chapters.

He often used to say, "The universe is always talking to us — sending us little messages, causing coincidences and serendipitous events, reminding us to stop, to look around, and to believe in something special, something more. But this special something isn't somewhere else. It's right where you are."

Be focused on the present moment and take action with full confidence in yourself.

REFERENCES

1. Decade of Healthy Ageing: Baseline Report, 14 January 2021, Global Report.

2. Older adults absorb protein less effectively: J. Brody, "Muscle Loss in Ageing Can Be Reversed," The New York Times, September 4, 2028, p. D5.

3. Chowdhury et al., "Association of Dietary Circulating and Supplement Fatty Acids."

4. Eighth Leading Cause of Death: C. Troeger et al., "Estimates of the Global, Regional, and National Morbidity, Mortality, and Aetiologies of Diarrhoea in 195 Countries: A Systematic Analysis for the Global Burden of Disease Study 2016," Lancet Infectious Diseases 18, no. 11 (2018): 1211-1228.

5. The 5 AM Club by Robin Sharma.

6. Peterson, T. (2021, December 26). https://www.healthyplace.com/self-help/self-help-information/what-mental-wellbeing-definition-and-examples.

7. TIME article New Age: Four Questions to Inner Peace by Jeffrey Ressner, Monday, December 11, 2000.

8. What is emotional well-being? 8 Ways to Improve Your Mental Health.

9. Approaches to Enhance Social Connection in Older Adults: An Integrative Review of Literature by Usar Suragarn, Ph.D., MSN, R.N., Debra Hain, Ph.D., APRN, ANP-BC, GNP-BC, FAANP, FAAN, Glenn Pfaff, MSN, R.N., Volume 1, Issue 3, September 2021, 100029.

DISCLAIMER

This book is for educational purposes only. Readers acknowledge that the author does not render legal, financial, medical, or professional advice. The content within this book has been derived from various sources. Please consult a licensed professional before attempting any techniques outlined in this book.

By reading this document, the reader agrees that under no circumstances is the author responsible for any direct or indirect losses incurred as a result of the use of the information contained within this document, including but not limited to errors, omissions, or inaccuracies.

Adherence to all applicable laws and regulations, including international, federal, state, and local governing professional licensing, business practices, advertising, and all other jurisdictions, is the sole responsibility of the purchaser or reader.

Neither the author nor the publisher assumes any responsibility or liability whatsoever on behalf of the purchaser or reader of these materials. Any perceived slight of any individual or organization is purely unintentional.

www.ingramcontent.com/pod-product-compliance
Lightning Source LLC
Chambersburg PA
CBHW051747250726
48659CB00001B/292